# Transcriptome Analysis

*Edited by Miroslav Blumenberg*

Published in London, United Kingdom

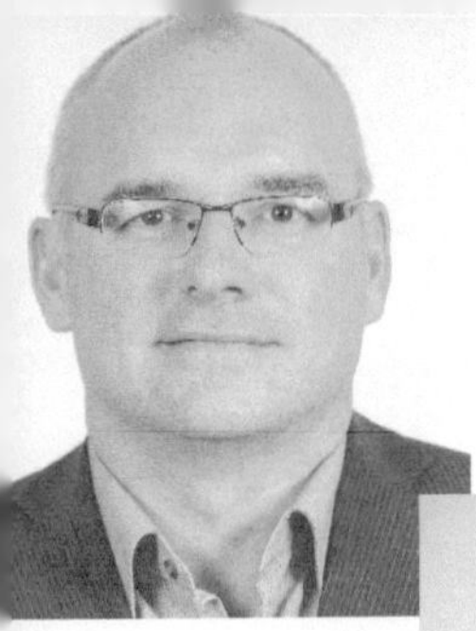
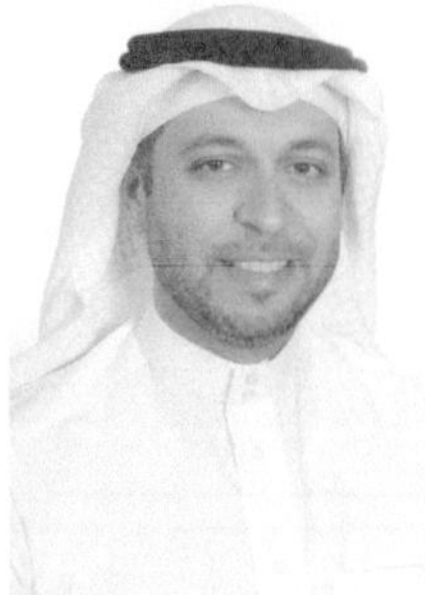
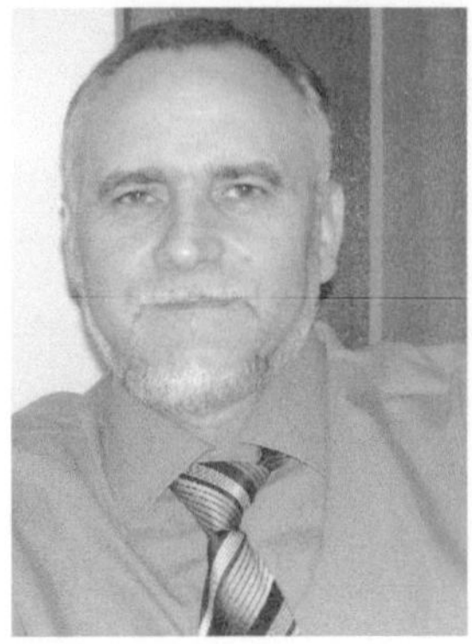
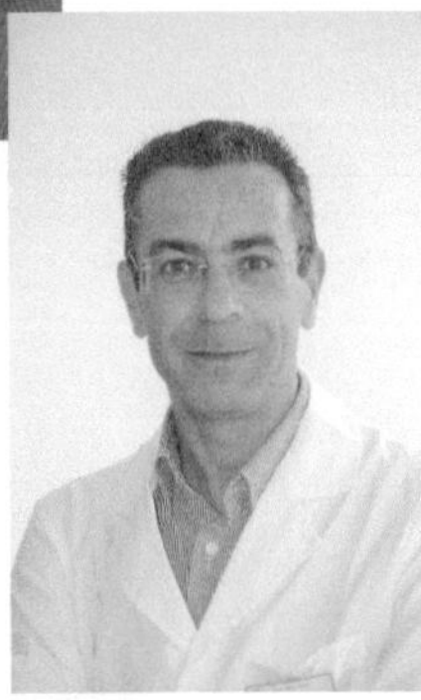
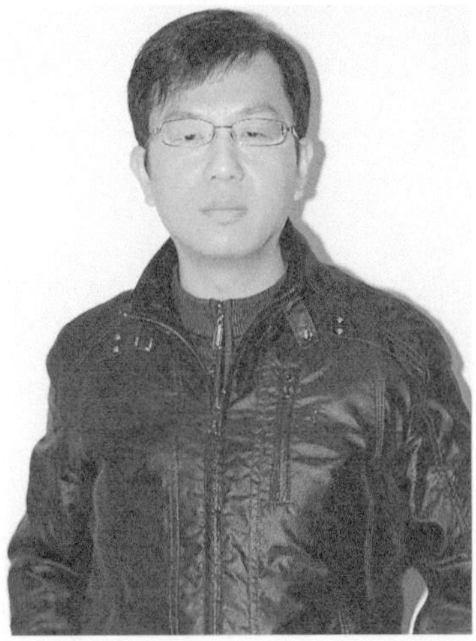
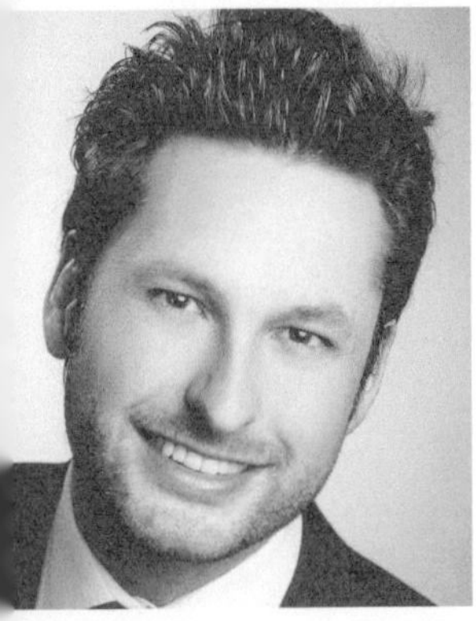
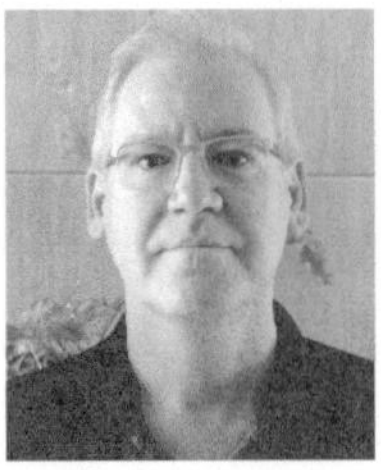

IntechOpen

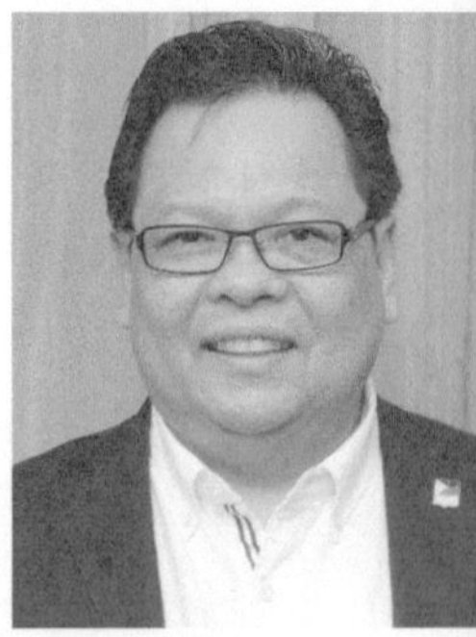
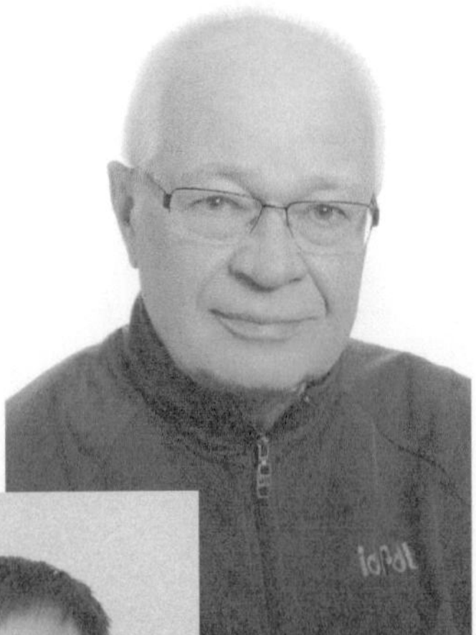
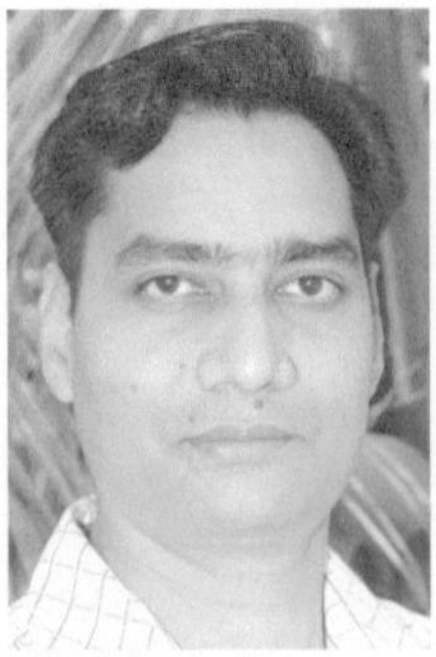
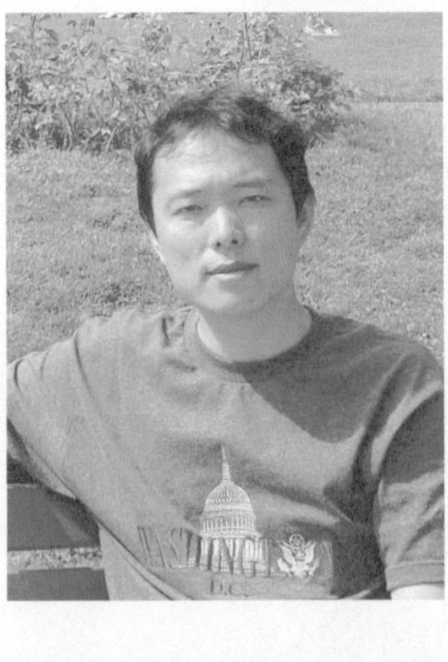
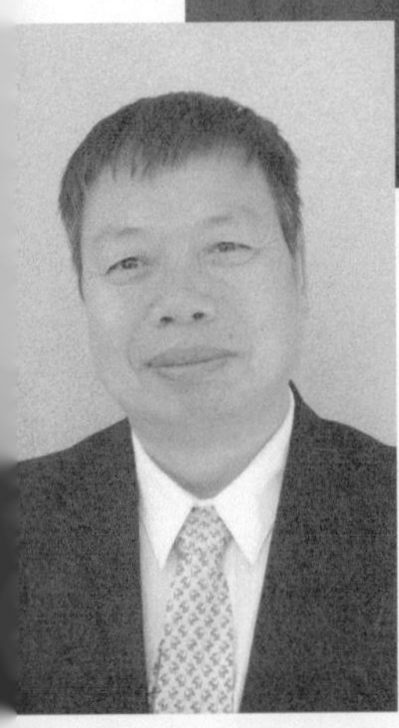
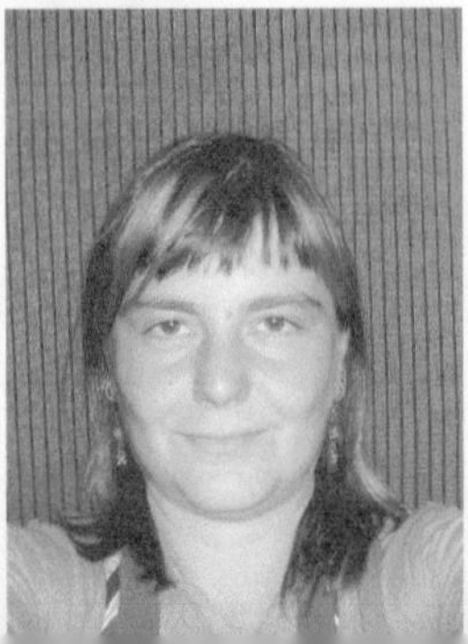

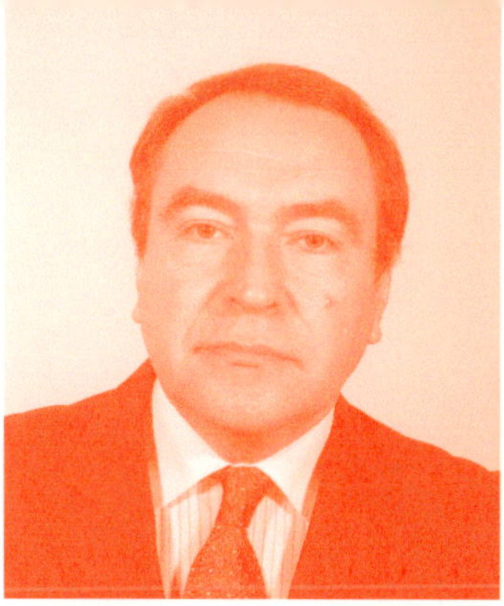

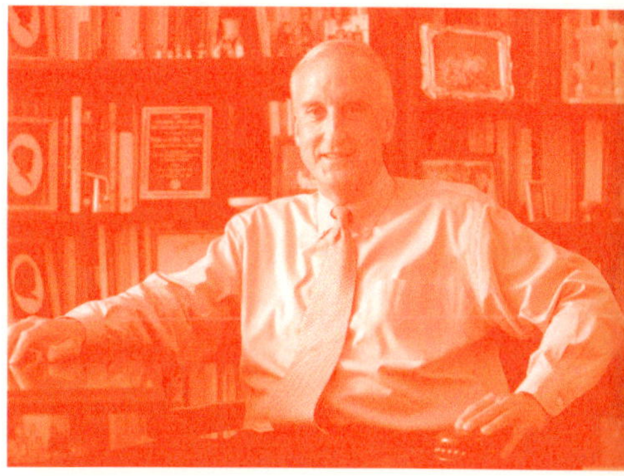

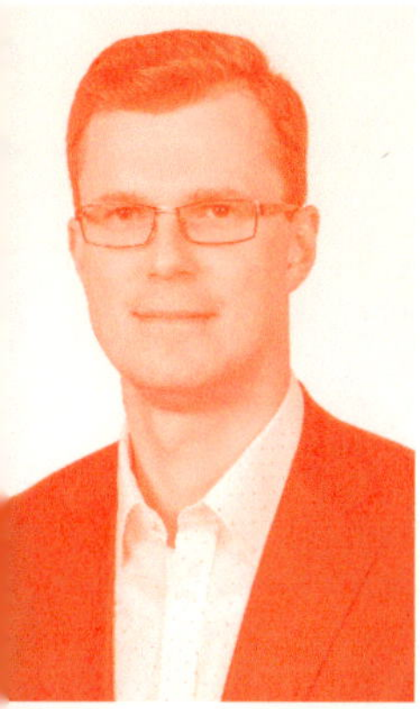

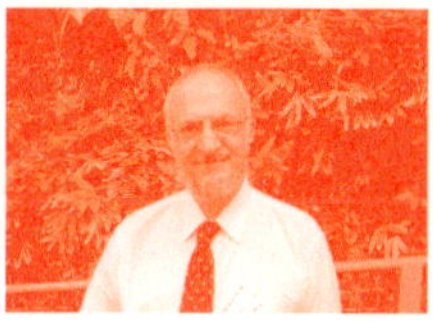

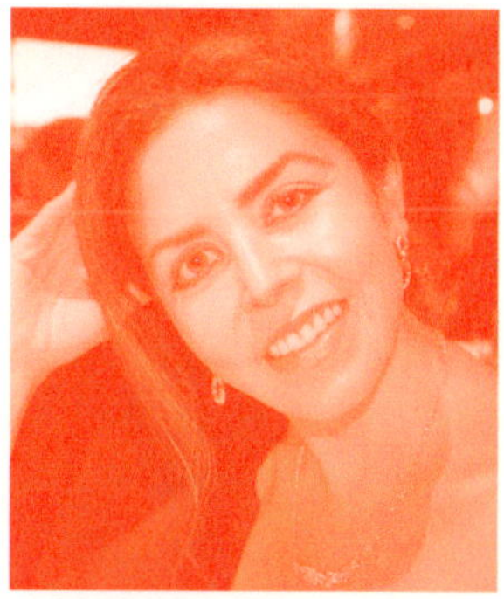

*Supporting open minds since 2005*

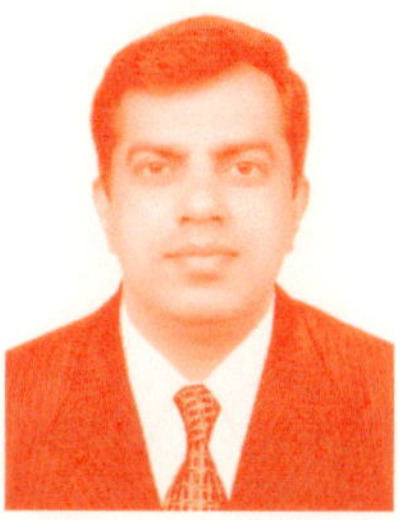

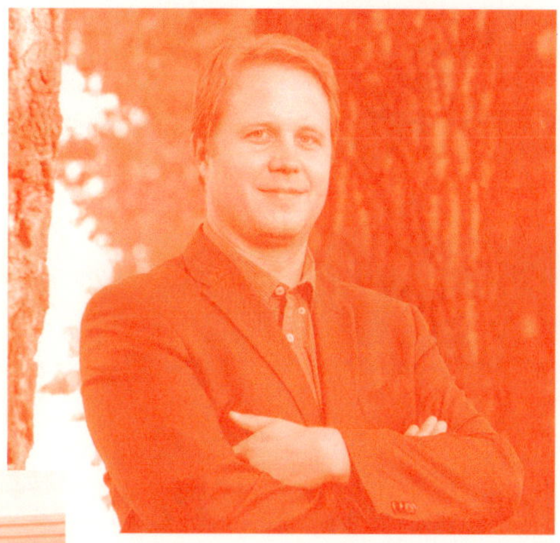

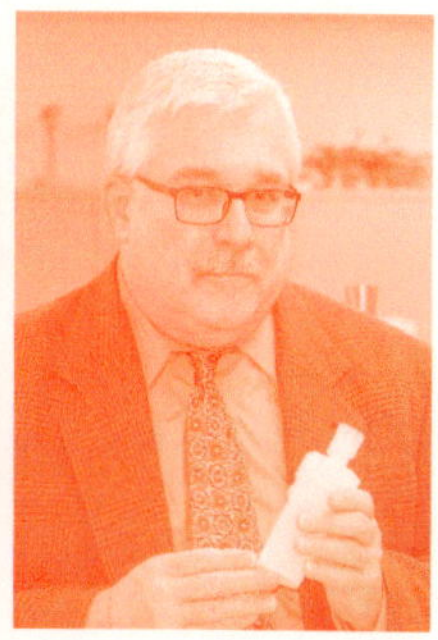

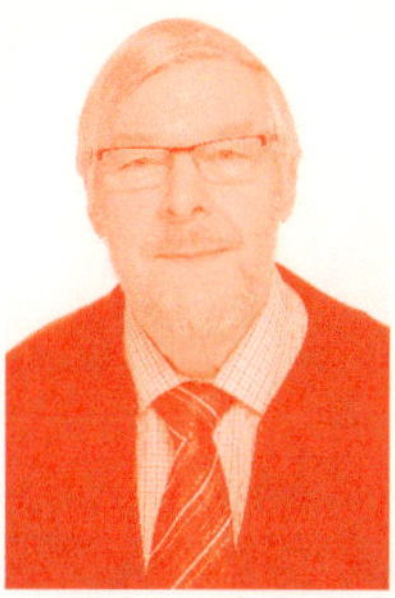

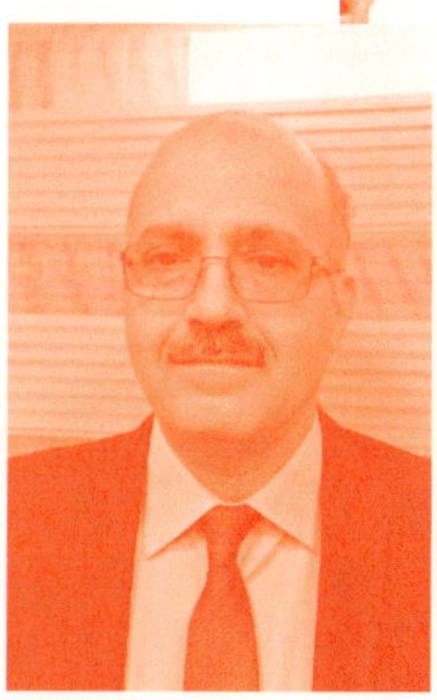

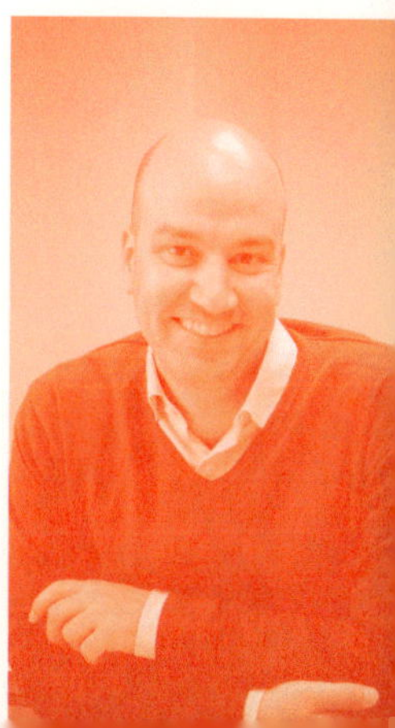

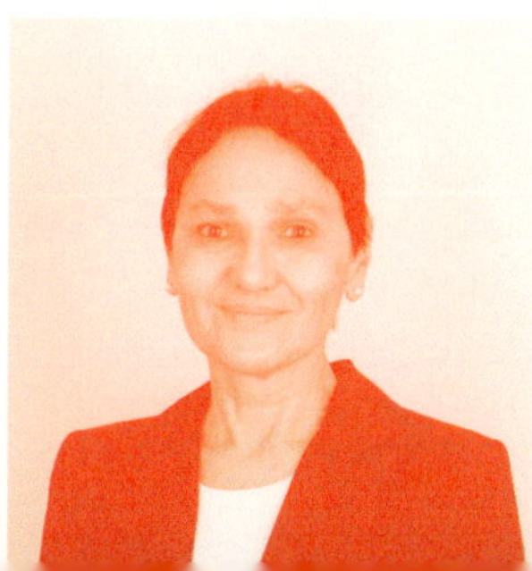

Transcriptome Analysis
http://dx.doi.org/10.5772/intechopen.77860
Edited by Miroslav Blumenberg

Contributors
Michael Sadovsky, Yulia Putintseva, Vladislav Biryukov, Maria Senashova, Chang Pyo Hong, Dong Jin Lee, Shinichi Hashimoto, Sadahiro Iwabuchi, Prasanta K. Dash, Ashutosh Kumar, Miroslav Blumenberg, Xiangyuan Wan, Ziwen Li



First published in London, United Kingdom, 2019 by IntechOpen
IntechOpen is the global imprint of INTECHOPEN LIMITED, registered in England and Wales, registration number: 11086078, 7th floor, 10 Lower Thames Street, London, EC3R 6AF, United Kingdom
Printed in Croatia

British Library Cataloguing-in-Publication Data
A catalogue record for this book is available from the British Library

Additional hard and PDF copies can be obtained from orders@intechopen.com

Transcriptome Analysis
Edited by Miroslav Blumenberg
p. cm.
Print ISBN 978-1-78984-327-9
Online ISBN 978-1-78984-328-6
eBook (PDF) ISBN 978-1-78985-263-9

For EU product safety concerns:
IN TECH d.o.o., Prolaz Marije Krucifikse Kozulić 3, 51000 Rijeka, Croatia, info@intechopen.com or visit our website at intechopen.com.

# Meet the editor

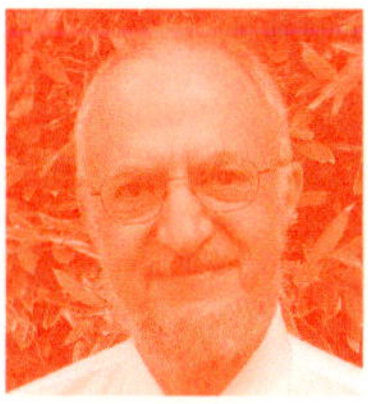

Miroslav Blumenberg, PhD, was born in Subotica and received his BSc in Belgrade, Yugoslavia. He completed his PhD at MIT in Organic Chemistry; he followed up his PhD with two postdoctoral study periods at Stanford University. Since 1983, he has been a faculty member of the RO Perelman Department of Dermatology, NYU School of Medicine, where he is a codirector of a training grant in cutaneous biology. Dr. Blumenberg's research is focused on the epidermis, expression of keratin genes, transcription profiling, keratinocyte differentiation, inflammatory diseases and cancers, and most recently the effects of the microbiome on skin. He has published more than 100 peer-reviewed research articles and graduated numerous PhD and postdoctoral students. Dr. Blumenberg lives in New York, USA, with his wife and two children.

# Contents

# Preface

Transcriptome analysis is the study of the transcriptome, of the complete set of RNA transcripts that are produced under specific circumstances, using high-throughput methods. Transcription profiling, which follows total changes in the behavior of a cell, is used throughout diverse areas of biomedical research, including diagnosis of disease, biomarker discovery, risk assessment of new drugs or environmental chemicals, etc. Transcription profiling can be applied to loss- and gain-of-function mutants to identify the changes associated with the mutant phenotype. Transcriptomics also allows the identification of pathways that respond to or ameliorate environmental stresses. RNA sequencing (RNA-Seq) detects all transcripts in a sample, including mRNAs as well as the regulatory siRNA and lncRNA transcripts. RNA-Seq can also identify disease-associated gene fusions, single nucleotide polymorphisms, and even allele-specific expression.

Transcriptome analysis is most commonly used to compare specific pairs of samples. The differences may be due to different external environmental conditions, for example, hormonal effects or toxins. More commonly, healthy and disease states are compared. In general, transcriptome analysis is a very powerful hypothesis-generating tool rather than a theory-proving one. Transcriptome analyses have become indispensable in basic research and translational and clinical studies.

In this volume, Dr. Pyo Hong discusses the role of long RNA sequences in transcriptome analysis. It should be noted that early RNA-Seq methods generated rather short reads, 35 to a few hundred nucleotides, and relied on massive redundancy to achieve required accuracy. Newer methods, which provide longer reads, have significant advantages, for example, in the analysis of previously not sequenced genomes. Such approaches need tailored software methods.

Dr. Shinichi describes next-generation single-cell sequencing technology developed by his team. It can be used for single-cell transcriptome analysis in tumor tissues. This is an extremely important area nowadays because it is clear that most tumors are heterogeneous. Identifying the transcriptome of tumor stem cells may lead to specific targeting of these cells. Alternatively, single-cell transcriptome analysis can help in defining the tumor-infiltrating immune cells, a critical component of immunotherapies. Dr. Shinichi and his team developed a microwell device that can be easily transported and is relatively cheaper than most other RNA-Seq methods, which will be essential for the widespread use of transcription analysis, especially in the developing world.

Dr. Prasanta presents transcriptome analysis applied to rice, one of world's most essential staple foods. Rice production and yield are critically affected by environmental factors, including drought, flooding, high salinity, extreme temperatures, nutrient and mineral availability, toxins and pollutants, etc. Because of the complexity of influences on crop yield, it is essential to define the intricate regulatory gene networks and their signaling pathways involved in stress responses. High-throughput RNA-Seq data have provided an abundance of transcriptome data on rice. RNA-Seq provides data regarding not only coding mRNAs but also noncoding RNAs, components of regulatory gene networks involved in the stress response. These results may enable more optimal cultivating conditions and help to develop new tolerant varieties of rice.

Dr. Xiangyuan focused his studies on the reproductive systems of flowering plants, specifically the gene regulatory networks in anthers, the parts of the stamen that produce and contain pollen.

Prof. Sadovsky analyzed the coding sequences of few conifers, comparing the usage of triplet codons in cold-adjusted plants.

We can anticipate a greatly expanded usage of transcriptome analysis, especially when translated to the bedside, to provide better understanding and more specific diagnoses, enabling physicians to establish diagnoses quickly and reliably.

**Miroslav Blumenberg**
NYU School of Medicine,
USA

# Section 1

# Introduction

Chapter 1

# Introductory Chapter: Transcriptome Analysis

*Miroslav Blumenberg*

The central dogma of molecular biology describes the flow of genetic information from genes to functions of the cells and organisms. This comprises a two-step process: first, DNA, the permanent, heritable, genetic information repository, is transcribed by the RNA polymerase enzymes into RNA, a short-lasting information carrier; second, a subset of RNA, the messenger RNAs, mRNAs, are translated into protein. The **transcriptome,** then, is the complete set of all RNA molecules in a cell, a population of cells or in an organism.

Importantly, not all RNAs are translated into proteins, some serve a structural function, for example, rRNAs in the assembly of ribosomes, others are transporters, e.g., tRNAs, yet others serve regulatory functions, for example, the siRNAs, short interfering RNA, or lncRNAs, long non-coding RNAs; these are not translated into proteins [1]. However, these non-coding RNAs can and often do play roles in human diseases such as cancer, cardiovascular, and neurological disorders. While transcriptomics is most commonly applied to the mRNAs, the coding transcripts, transcriptomics also provides important data regarding content of the cell noncoding RNAs, including rRNA, tRNA, lncRNA, siRNA, and others. Specific approaches address the analysis of splice variant of the same gene in different tissues.

## 1. Transcriptome analysis

Transcriptome Analysis is the study of the transcriptome, of the complete set of RNA transcripts that are produced by the genome, under specific circumstances or in a specific cell, using high-throughput methods. Transcription profiling, which follows changes in behavior of a cell *in toto*, not of a single gene or just a few genes, is used throughout diverse areas of biomedical research, including disease diagnosis, biomarker discovery, risk assessment of new drugs or environmental chemicals etc. Transcription profiling can be applied to loss- and gain-of-function mutants to identify the changes associated with the mutant phenotype. The transcriptomic techniques have been particularly useful in identifying the functions of genes. Transcriptomics also allows identification of pathways that respond to or ameliorate environmental stresses. RNA-Seq can also identify disease-associated gene fusions, single nucleotide polymorphisms and even allele-specific expression.

## 2. Uses of transcriptome analysis

Transcriptome Analysis is most commonly used to compare specific pairs of samples. The differences may be due to different external environmental conditions, e.g., hormonal effects or toxins. More commonly, healthy and disease states



IntechOpen

are compared. For example, in cancer, transcriptomics analyses address classification, the mechanisms of pathogenesis and even outcome prediction. Transcriptome studies can classify cancer beyond anatomical location and histopathology. Outcome predictions can establish gene-based benchmarks to predict tumor prognosis and therapy response. These approaches are already in use for personalized medicine, individualized cancer patient therapies.

Organisms and tissues at various stages of development can be molecularly characterized. The transcriptomes of stem cells help to understand the processes of cellular differentiation or embryonic development. Because of its very broad approach transcriptome analysis is a great source for identifying targets for treatment.

## 2.1 Methodologies

The early approach to study whole transcriptomes used microarrays, a set of defined sequences arranged on a solid substrate [2]. Microarrays almost exclusively represented mRNAs, that is, genes that are translated into proteins.

Nowadays the microarray approach is supplanted by high-throughput RNA sequencing, RNA-Seq, which detects all transcripts in a sample, including the regulatory siRNA and lncRNA transcripts [3]. In this methodology, the bulk RNA is extracted from the sample and copied into stable double-stranded copy DNA, ds-cDNA, which is then sequenced using various sequencing methods [4]. The sequences obtained are aligned to reference genome sequences, available in data banks, to identify which genes are transcribed. Quantitatively, the results provide the expression levels for the transcribed genes. Compared to microarrays, RNA-Seq can measure both the low-abundance and high-abundance RNAs over a five orders of magnitude range and, importantly, RNA-Seq requires much less starting material (nanograms vs. micrograms and even as little as 50 pg) [5]. This made possible analyses of transcriptomes in a single cell, a great advance over bulk tissue RNA analyses [6]. RNA-seq can be used to identify alternative splicing, novel transcripts, and fusion genes (**Table 1**).

In principle, the assembly of RNA-Seq reads is not dependent on reference genomes and can be used for gene expression studies of poorly characterized species with limited genomic resources. It can also be used to identify novel protein coding regions in sequenced genomes. RNA-seq can be performed using many next-generation sequencing platforms, however, each platform has its own requirements of sample preparation and the instrument design.

| Method | Read length | Accuracy | Reads per run | Time per run | Cost per 1 million bp | Advantages | Disadvantages |
|---|---|---|---|---|---|---|---|
| Single-molecule real-time sequencing<br>Pacific Biosciences | >100,000 bases | 87% | 500,000 per Sequel SMRT cell<br>10 to 20 gigabases | 30 minutes to 20 hours | $0.05–$0.08 | Fast. | Expensive. |
| Ion semiconductor<br>Ion Torrent sequencing | Up to 600 bp | 99.60% | up to 80 million | 2 hours | 1 | Less expensive equipment. Fast. | Homopolymer errors. |
| Pyrosequencing<br>454 Life Sciences | Up to 700 bp | 99.90% | 1 million | 24 hours | $10 | Long read size. Fast. | Runs are expensive.<br>Homopolymer errors. |
| Sequencing by synthesis<br>Illumina | 50–600 bp | 99.90% | 1 Million to 2.5 billion | 1 to 11 days | $0.05 to $0.15 | High sequence yield. | Expensive equipment.<br>Requires high DNA concentrations. |
| Combinatorial probe anchor synthesis<br>cPAS- BGI/MGI | 35-300 bp | 99.90% | 50 to 1300M per flow cell | 1 to 9 days | $0.035- $0.12 | | |
| Sequencing by ligation<br>SOLiD sequencing | 50+50 bp | 99.90% | 1.2 to 1.4 billion | 1 to 2 weeks | $0.13 | Low cost per base. | Slower.<br>Issues with palindromic sequences. |
| Nanopore Sequencing | Up to 500 kb | 92–97% | Up to 500 kb | 1 min to 48 hrs | Depends | Portable. | Lower throughput.<br>Lower accuracy. |
| Chain termination Sanger sequencing | 400 to 900 bp | 99.90% | N/A | 20 minutes to 3 hours | $2,400 | Useful for many applications. | Time consuming lab bench steps |

**Table 1.**
*Comparison of RNA-seq methodologies.*

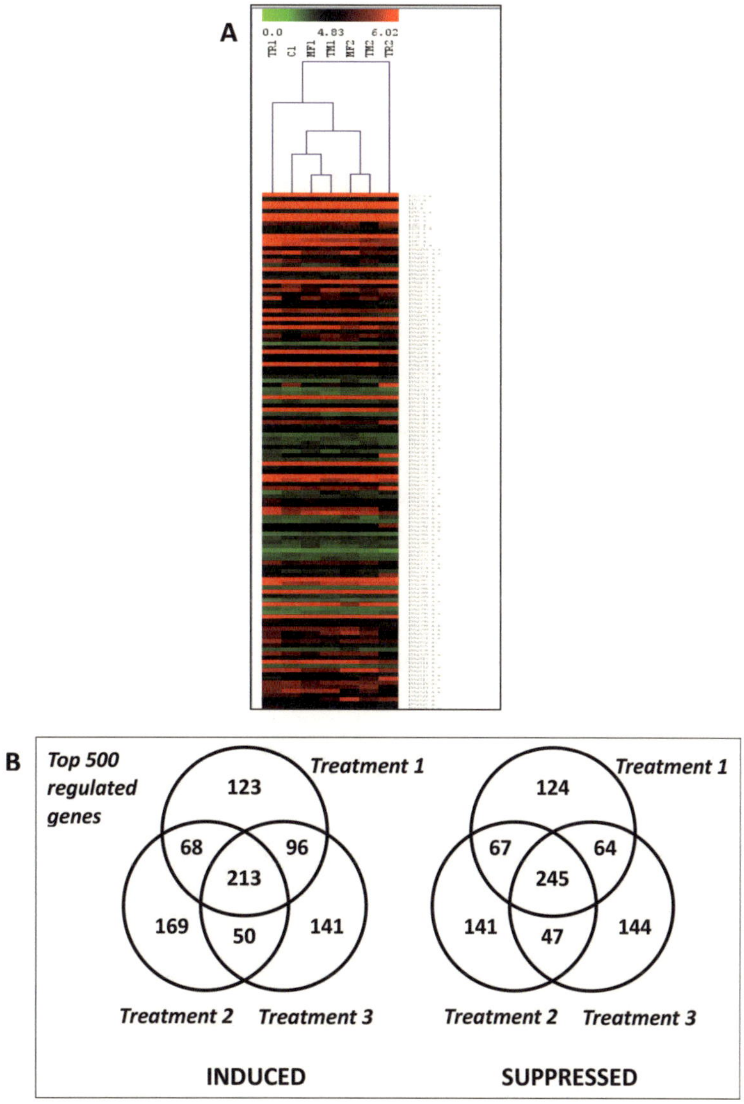


**Figure 1.**
*Graphic representations of transcriptome analysis data. (A) Heat map with clustering tree. (B) Venn diagrams of regulated genes.*

## 2.2 Data analysis, repositories and presentation

Improved sequencing technologies necessitated improved data analysis methods to deal with the increased volume of data produced by each transcriptome experiment. Importantly, the results are deposited into transcriptome databases, essential tools for transcriptome analysis. For example Gene Expression Omnibus, www.ncbi.nml.nih.gov, contains millions of transcription profiling experiments. Such data have potential applications beyond the original aims of an experiment. Typical outputs include quantitative tables of the transcript levels. This requires specific analysis algorithms, often specific to the methodology used. There are software packages to bridge data from disparate methodologies, to identify groups of similar expressed genes, or differentially expressed functionally significant regulatory or metabolic pathways.

The results of transcriptomic analyses are graphically often presented as heat maps, a system of color-coding that represents different levels of expression of given genes in different samples (**Figure 1A**). Such presentations also frequently display a clustering of samples, this helps to identify samples with similar gene expression. Another common graphical presentation uses Venn diagrams, which count the transcripts which are equivalently regulated in multiple samples (**Figure 1B**).

Transcriptome analyses have become indispensable in basic research, translational, and clinical studies. In general, transcriptome analysis is a very powerful hypothesis-generating tool, more than a theory proving one.

## 3. Specific example: transcriptome analysis applied to human skin

Easily accessible, skin was among the first targets analyzed using 'omics' and dermatology embraced the approaches very early [7]. A classic example of coordinated transcriptional regulation was observed in cultured fibroblasts after serum stimulation [2]. Serum addition causes not only rapid recommencement of the cell cycle but, characteristically a wound-healing response, a physiological role of fibroblasts in wound healing [8]. Transcriptional responses of epidermal keratinocytes to UV light, hormones, vitamins, infections, inflammatory and immunomodulating cytokines, toxins and allergens have been characterized, as were the changes associated with epidermal differentiation [9, 10].

The expression signatures that define the various cell types in human skin, were used to define 20 specific gene signatures, including those for keratinocytes, melanocytes, endothelia, adipocytes, immune cells, hair follicles, sebaceous, sweat, and apocrine glands. This resource provided a resource named SkinSig, which was then used to analyze 18 skin conditions, providing in-context interpretation of, for example, influx in immune cells in inflammation or differentiation changes in disorders of cornification [11].

In the future we can anticipate a greatly expanded usage of transcriptome analysis. Translated to the bedside, it can provide better understanding and more specific diagnoses of diseases. This, of course, requires additional advances in the technology, both in the lab-bench components reducing the costs and guaranteeing reproducibility and accuracy, as well as in the computer-based components, algorithms that enable physicians to establish diagnosis quickly and reliably. In a generation, this approach will become routine.

## Author details

Miroslav Blumenberg
NYU School of Medicine, USA

*Address all correspondence to: miroslav.blumenberg@nyulangone.org

## References

[1] Botchkareva NV. The molecular revolution in cutaneous biology: Noncoding RNAs: New molecular players in dermatology and cutaneous biology. The Journal of Investigative Dermatology. 2017;**137**(5):e105-e111. DOI: 10.1016/j.jid.2017.02.001. PMID: 28411840

[2] Iyer VR, Eisen MB, Ross DT, Schuler G, Moore T, Lee JC, et al. The transcriptional program in the response of human fibroblasts to serum. Science. 1999;**283**(5398):83-87. PMID: 9872747

[3] Bayega A, Fahiminiya S, Oikonomopoulos S, Ragoussis J. Current and future methods for mRNA analysis: A drive toward single molecule sequencing. Methods in Molecular Biology. 2018;**1783**:209-241. DOI: 10.1007/978-1-4939-7834-2_11. PMID: 29767365

[4] Zhang H, He L, Cai L. Transcriptome sequencing: RNA-Seq. Methods in Molecular Biology. 2018;**1754**:15-27. DOI: 10.1007/978-1-4939-7717-8_2. PMID: 29536435

[5] Shanker S, Paulson A, Edenberg HJ, Peak A, Perera A, Alekseyev YO, et al. Evaluation of commercially available RNA amplification kits for RNA sequencing using very low input amounts of total RNA. Journal of Biomolecular Techniques. 2015 April;**26**(1):4-18. DOI: 10.7171/jbt.15-2601-001. PMC 4310221. PMID 25649271

[6] Stegle O, Teichmann SA, Marioni JC. Computational and analytical challenges in single-cell transcriptomics. Nature Reviews Genetics. 2015;**16**(3):133-145. DOI: 10.1038/nrg3833. PMID: 25628217

[7] Mimoso C, Lee DD, Zavadil J, Tomic-Canic M, Blumenberg M. Analysis and meta-analysis of transcriptional profiling in human epidermis. Methods in Molecular Biology. 2014;**1195**:61-97. DOI: 10.1007/7651_2013_60

[8] Eming SA, Martin P, Tomic-Canic M. Wound repair and regeneration: Mechanisms, signaling, and translation. Science Translational Medicine. 2014;**6**(265):265sr6. DOI: 10.1126/scitranslmed.3009337. PMID: 25473038

[9] Blumenberg M. Skinomics: Past, present and future for diagnostic microarray studies in dermatology. Expert Review of Molecular Diagnostics. 2013;**13**(8):885-894. DOI: 10.1586/14737159.2013.846827. PMID: 24151852

[10] Santoro S, Lopez ID, Lombardi R, Zauli A, Osiceanu AM, Sorosina M, et al. Laser capture microdissection for transcriptomic profiles in human skin biopsies. BMC Molecular Biology. 2018;**19**(1):7. DOI: 10.1186/s12867-018-0108-5. PMID: 29921228 PMCID: PMC6009967

[11] Shih BB, Nirmal AJ, Headon DJ, Akbar AN, Mabbott NA, Freeman TC. Derivation of marker gene signatures from human skinand their use in the interpretation of the transcriptional changes associated with dermatological disorders. The Journal of Pathology. 2017;**241**(5):600-613. DOI: 10.1002/path.4864. Epub 2017 Feb 24. PMID: 28008606 PMCID: PMC5363360

## Section 2

# Tumor Transcriptome

Chapter 2

# Single-Cell Transcriptome Analysis in Tumor Tissues

*Sadahiro Iwabuchi and Shinichi Hashimoto*


## Abstract

The tumor microenvironment is comprised of cancer cells and their surroundings, including various normal cells and non-cellular components, and each tumor tissue has a distinctive microenvironment. Cancer progression is affected by different microenvironmental states, such as the heterogeneity of infiltrating immune cells. Therefore, it is necessary to understand the complex cell-to-cell interactions associated with tumor developmental stages in different tissues. Recent revolution of single-cell RNA sequencing technology can uncover the tumor microenvironment diversity. We have developed a novel strategy of single-cell transcriptome analysis: next generation 1-cell sequencing (Nx1-seq) technology, and it allows for profiling of thousands of single cells from tumor tissue. Our microwell with cell bar-code beads device can detect genes with high sensitivity, and it is easily transported anywhere without any other dedicated devices. Further, the developmental cost is relatively cheaper than other single-cell RNA sequencing methods. In this study, we introduce representative application of the single-cell RNA sequencing technique in gynecological cancers, and we show the result of Nx1-seq application in human endometrioid adenocarcinoma tissue.


**Keywords:** tumor microenvironment, single-cell transcriptome analysis, Nx1-seq

## 1. Introduction

Tumor tissues are aggregates of various cell populations, and each single cell or cell population plays an important role for cancer progression and regression. The representative cell populations of the tumor microenvironment are cancer cells, surrounding normal cells, and infiltrated immune cells of all types. Anticancer agents and immune checkpoint blockers, such as programmed death receptor-1 (PD-1) and its ligand, have been widely used in patients, and the curative effect is great. However, for many patients, these treatments are ineffective because the minor cell populations escape the immune system. Therefore, a deeper understanding of the tumor microenvironment immunology will be critical for immunotherapy to become a standard therapy. In addition, it is important to clarify patient and tumor-dependent cell phenotypes by gene expression analysis because the composition and functions of the tumor microenvironment are heterogeneous between cancers and patients.

Previous gene expression measurements have been performed on bulk samples. Conventional bulk-based RNA sequencing or microarrays alone or in combination with flow cytometry can provide a full view of all gene expression, and it is useful to investigate the tumor microenvironment. However, a blended gene expression analysis might mask the minor cell population, which may be the origin of tumor progression. To overcome this problem, RNA sequencing methods that can analyze mRNA expression at the single-cell level from thousands of individual cells are required. The fundamentally necessary approaches of single-cell RNA sequencing are: (1) single-cell isolation with a high survival rate, (2) cell lysis to obtain mRNA, (3) conversion of mRNA into cDNA, (4) specific amplification of cDNA, (5) cDNA fragmentation process, and (6) creation of high-quality sequencing libraries. After single-cell isolation, there are some innovate single-cell transcriptome analysis methods (e.g., CEL-seq [1], Quartz-seq [2], Quartz-seq2 [3], Smart-seq [4], Drop-seq [5], iDrop RNA sequencing [6], Cyto-Seq [7], automated microwell-based RNA sequencing [8], and our next generation 1-cell sequencing; Nx1-seq [9]), and every method uses oligo-dT primers containing cell-specific bar-codes, which tag cDNA from single cells.

Although cell number, tissue volume analyzed, analysis sensitivity, and overall cost for creating libraries are completely different, any methods with an efficient data analysis procedure would be particularly useful to understand cellular heterogeneity and to identify rare cell populations. For example, six prominent single-cell RNA sequencing methods: CEL-seq2, Drop-seq, MARS-seq, SCRB-seq, Smart-seq, and Smart-seq2 have been compared in mouse embryonic stem cells [10]. If single-cell transcriptome analysis were performed in a limited number of cells or small tissue volume, SCREB-seq and MARS-seq will have better sensitivity. Yet, Smart-seq2 may detect the highest number of genes per cell with amplification noise. Drop-seq is a preferable and more cost-effective method for large numbers of cells with low sequencing depth. In terms of the number of reads per cell and genes, we also compared our Nx1-seq and Drop-seq, and it revealed similar sensitivity [9]. Recently, another microwell-based RNA sequencing has been developed [11], and this is a simple, high-throughput, and low-cost device. The principle of their device is similar to Cyto-Seq and Nx1-seq, but the differences are the beads material and the loading order of single cells and beads to the microwell. They have attempted to construct a "mouse cell atlas" by using over 50 mouse tissues, organs, and cell cultures. One of the reasons they can analyze a large sample amount is the low-cost device without any expensive, exclusive apparatus and kits for capturing mRNA from a single cell. Previously, a detailed description of each method was thoroughly reviewed [12]; yet, innovate new technologies for single-cell RNA sequencing are still to be developed. We also continue improving our Nx1-seq device progressively.

## 2. Single-cell transcriptome analysis for cancer tissues

To find new molecular targets for a cancer prognosis prediction method, it requires an understanding of the single-cell level transcriptome heterogeneity in tumor tissues and their microenvironment. Bulk-based RNA sequencing may also contribute to development of new minimally invasive monitoring of circulating tumor cells or cancer gene-transferred macrophages and lymphoid cells. If the targeted cancer antigen and/or cell surface protein were held in small cell populations, the intensity signal of the gene expression would be weak. In this case, single cell transcriptome analysis is a useful tool to identify the small cell population and obtain all of the gene information in this population. In the next chapter, we describe our Nx1-seq methods in detail and show a representative Nx1-seq application in human endometrioid adenocarcinoma tissue. At this time, there are no reports about single-cell transcriptome analysis for endometrioid adenocarcinoma, except our research [9]. Here, we briefly summarize recent applications of single-cell RNA sequencing in one of the major gynecological cancers, breast cancer.

Chung et al. conducted single-cell transcriptome analysis for 11 primary tumors and 2 metastatic lymph nodes from 11 patients, representing 4 breast cancer subtypes [13]. It clearly displayed the carcinoma and tumor-infiltrating immune cells population using the 10–17 μm integrated fluidic circuit mRNA sequencing chip in the $C_1$™ Single-Cell Auto Prep System of Fluidigm®. The $C_1$™ integrate fluidic circuit is an integrated microfluidic system that can automatically isolate individual cells from suspended cells. Subsequently, cell lysis buffer is automatically applied to individual cells to capture mRNA. It takes 5 h to make sequence-ready libraries from isolated cells, and the operation is simple [14]. The authors demonstrated that many T cells with high cytokine and chemokine expression were observed in three triple negative breast cancers (TNBC), and their phenotypes were regulatory T cells (two out of three patients) and another one was exhaustion and cytotoxicity signatures [13]. This result indicates that immune checkpoint blockers may be effective in the patient.

Recently, single-cell transcriptome analysis using 10X Genomics Chromium was reported in breast cancer [15, 16]. Cazet et al. investigated the anti-tumor inhibitor effects in a mouse tumor model, in terms of changes in the gene expression profiles of each cell population [15]. Tumor development and progression were associated with stiffness of the extracellular matrix, and collagen density in the tumor-stromal interface was reduced by small molecule inhibitor of smoothened (SMO) treatment. They also showed that the chemotherapy significantly slowed tumor growth and reduced the frequency of metastatic disease in xenograft models of human TNBC. In another article, an infiltrating T cell population in breast cancer was classified from 123 patients, and it demonstrated the importance of qualitative identification of $CD8^+$ T cell subtypes [16]. $CD8^+$ $CD103^+$ T cells contained features of read tissue-resident memory, including high granzyme B, PD-1, and cytotoxic T lymphocyte (associated) antigen 4 (CTLA-4), rather than $CD8^+$ $CD103^-$ T cells, meaning that these are target cells for immune checkpoint brokers.

The above representative reports using single-cell read transcriptome analysis were well analyzed, but we speculate that the cost for creating a sequence library per sample using commercially available device-dependent kits may be expensive. Many samples should be analyzed in a clinical study because the observed microenvironment heterogeneity is patient-, malignant-, or organ-dependent. In addition, if characterization of tumor gene expression profiling was recognized according to the individual's region or country, it should be performed locally because fresh samples, not frozen ones, are better to analyze for RNA sequencing. From this standpoint, a device with low-cost, in high sensitivity, and easy performance is recommended.

## 3. Nx1-seq

The major component of Nx1-seq (next generation 1-cell sequencing) consists of bar-code beads and a specifically processed microwell. In this chapter, we describe these devices in further detail.

### 3.1 Bar-code beads

Oligonucleotides on beads have the following sequence: (1) "root array" is used as a priming site for subsequent PCR; (2) "cell bar-code" allocates 12 bp of oligonucleotide to identify cells, and the bar-code has $4^{12}$ = 16,777,216 various patterns; (3) "UMI" (a unique molecular identifier) has 8 bp of oligonucleotide to eliminate gene duplication bias and improve signal/noise ratio by PCR, meaning that 1-cell bar-code has 1 UMI; and (4) "poly-dT" array consists of 25 bp oligo dT sequences for capturing polyadenylated mRNA. The bar-code beads ("root"-"cell bar-code"-"UMI"-"poly-dT") were made by following a modified instruction manual for the GS Junior Titanium emulsion PCR Kit (Lib-L) from Roche® Applied Science or synthesized by ChemGenes Corporation (Wilmington, MA, USA) with additional annealing and ligation of the poly-dT array in our laboratory. The detailed method for generating bar-code beads using the emulsion PCR kit is described in our previous report [9]. We could get randomly synthesized various "cell bar-code" inserted bar-code beads, and the beads were washed with Low TE buffer (10 mM Tris-HCl pH 8.0, 0.1 mM EDTA pH 8.0) and stored at −20°C until use.

### 3.2 Microwell slide

The microwell plate was prepared using polydimethylsiloxane (PDMS) and was cut 2 × 2 × 2 cm using cutting dies (Noda Co. Ltd., Osaka, Japan) which contained 1.3–1.6 × $10^5$ microwells. The size of one microwell was 25 ± 3 μm diameter, 40 ± 8 μm height, 20 ± 9 ρL capacity (column-shape), and the distance between microwells was 5 μm (YODAKA CO., Ltd., Kanagawa, Japan). If the size of the target cell was not between 15 and 25 μm, the diameter and height sizes were easily adjusted. The PDSM microwell plate was placed in an oxygen plasma chamber for hydrophilic processing because PDMS is a hydrophobic material. The microwell plate was quickly set into the Nunc™ Lab-Tek™ Chamber slide system (Thermo Fisher Scientific, Waltham, MA, USA), and bar-code beads were applied to the microwell plate. If the expected number of cells obtained from the tumor tissue was <1 × $10^5$ cells, the PDMS microwell was cut ~1/4 or 1/2 of its size and set into the appropriate Nunc™ Lab-Tek™ Chamber slide system (**Figure 1**). The PDMS microwell plate was kept at 4°C, meaning that the Nx1-seq device can be stored until use.

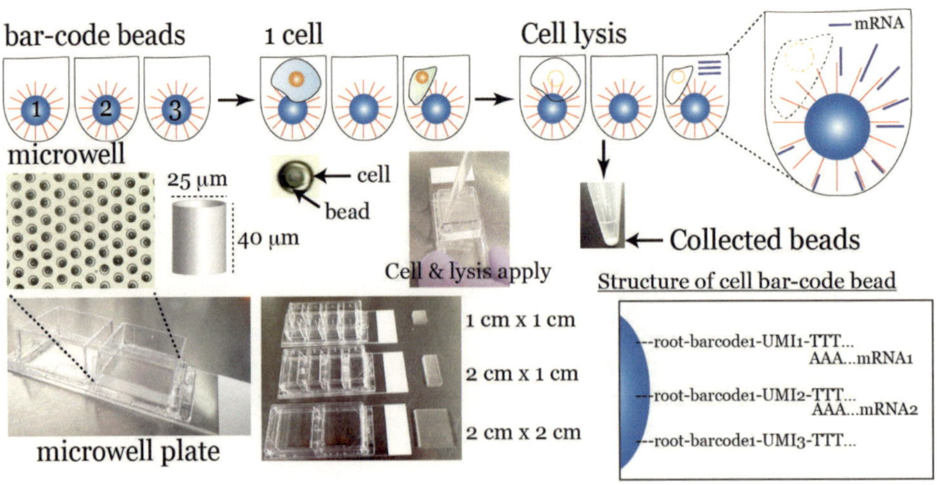


**Figure 1.**
*Schematic drawings of Nx1-seq. Cell bar-code beads (see the structure of cell bar-code bead) were filled into microwells, and an adequate number of single cells was applied. Cells were dissolved in lysis buffer, and mRNA from the cell was captured by cell bar-code beads in each microwell. After cellular lysis, all beads were collected into a single tube. Images of the microwell plate show that our device had some variations for differences of the number of applied cells.*

### 3.3 Lysis of cells

After single cell isolation, ~1–2 × $10^5$ cells mixed with 3.7 mL of cold PBS were applied to PDMS microwell plate (2 × 2 × 2 cm) and put the cover without entering a bubble. The microwell plate was put on ice for 10–15 min, which let the cells settle into the microwell by gravity. About 5% of whole microwells were filled with single cells according to Poisson distribution. The solution was removed from the microwell plate, and 1 mL of fresh cold PBS was gently applied. The washing process was repeated by 3–4 times. The reagent composition of 1 mL of cell lysis buffer was; 2 mg of *N*-Lauroylsarcosine sodium salt, 200 μL of 1 M Tris-HCl pH 7.5, 40 μL of 0.5 M EDTA pH 8.0, 750 μL of deionized water, 50 μL of 1 M dithiothreitol solution. The microwell plate was put on a microscopy, and we found the microwell which contains only cell without bar-code bead, then PBS was removed and 1 mL of cell lysis buffer was gently applied from the corner of the microwell. Most cells were getting to dissolve within 1–3 min, but it kept for 8 min. The cell lysis buffer was removed carefully and washing buffer (200 mM Tris-HCl pH 7.5, 20 mM EDTA, 50 mM DTT, 0.2% *N*-Lauroylsarcosine sodium salt, 2% Ficoll) was added. Conversion of mRNA into cDNA was done by SuperScript™ II or IV Reverse Transcriptase (Thermo Fisher Scientific).

## 4. Nx1-seq application to human endometrioid adenocarcinoma tissues

Previously, we reported the application of Nx1-seq to human endometrioid adenocarcinoma (EA) tissues [9]. Here, we summarize the result shortly. EA tissues were removed from the myometrial infiltration side (M-side) and endometrial side (E-side). Myometrial invasion is an independent prognostic parameter of EA, and invasion is correlated with the risk of metastasis to the lymph nodes. Single-cell analysis in each side revealed that EA had six cancer (cluster #0, 1, 2, 3, 5, 6), two macrophage (#4, 8), and one T cell population (#7) (**Figure 2A**). To analyze the sequencing data, we used Seurat software (http://satijalab.org/seurat/), which is an open tool for analyzing single-cell genomics in R (http://www.R-project.org/). As shown in **Figure 2B**, the distribution of cancer cells on the E-side and M-side differed, and the majority of the macrophage cluster (#4) was on the M-side. The number of infiltrating macrophages was not different between sides (**Figure 2C**), but macrophage specificity was more cytotoxic T lymphocytes (CTL)-like on the M-side. Macrophages on the M-side had higher expression of inflammatory chemokines, C-X-C motif chemokine ligand 3 and 8 (*CXCL3* and *CXCL8*) and NF-κ-B inhibitorα (*NFKBIA*) (**Figure 2D**). The proportion of macrophages expressing the inflammatory factors *CCL5*, *IL10* and *IL6* did not differ among the two sides (data not shown). It has been widely believed that many cells expressing some malignancy-related genes exist on the M-side; however, our previous result showed that cancer cells on the E-side were highly malignant when compared to those on the M-side.

In addition, a cancer stem-like cell population was also higher on the E-side (e.g., the ratio of *SOX2*$^+$ cells on E-side vs. M-side was 17 vs. 6%, respectively) [9]. These data reveal that cells with high malignant potential (HMP) are present at the same site of cancer tissue (E-side) in EA. To confirm our hypothesis, we focused on the ubiquitin C-terminal hydrolase L1 (*UCHL1*) gene. Protein ubiquitination or de-ubiquitination regulates cell growth, differentiation, transcription, and tumor prognosis. The function of *UCHL1* in neurodegenerative disorders, particularly in Alzheimer's disease and Parkinson's disease has been reported, and decreased

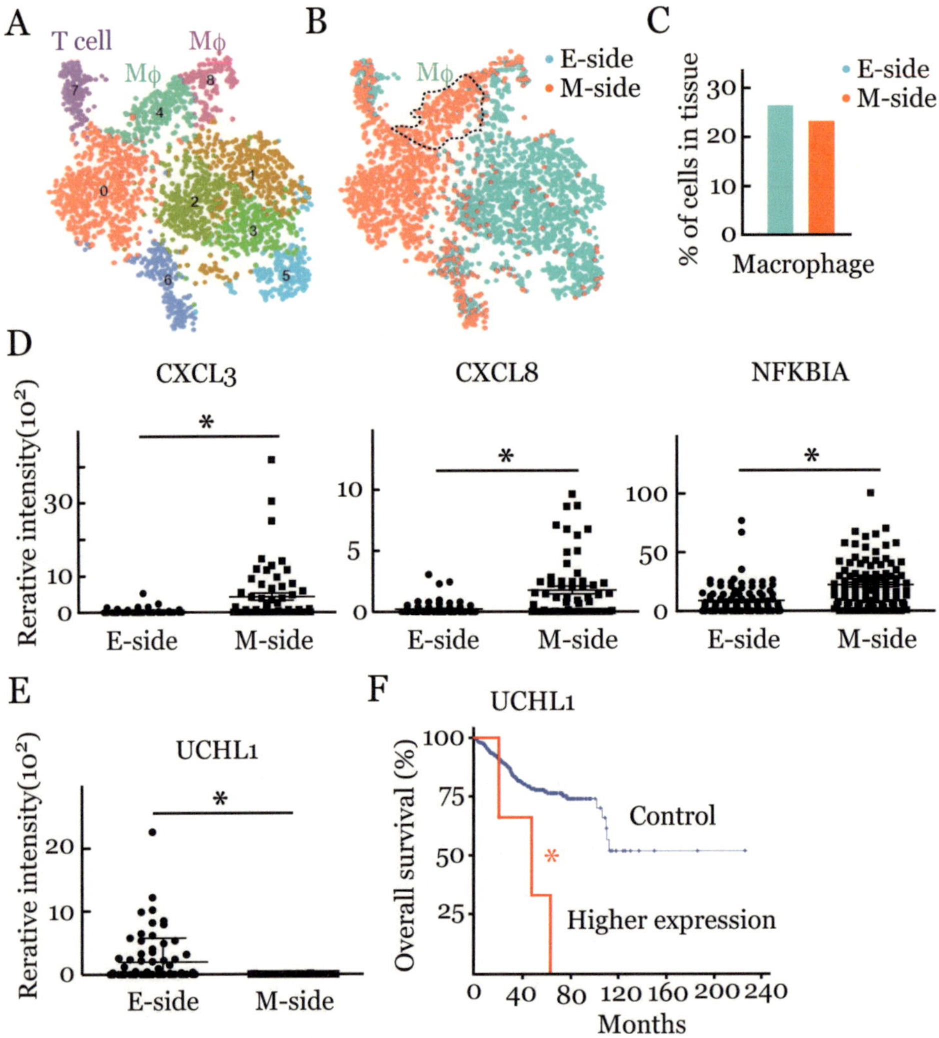


**Figure 2.**

*Clustering of human endometrioid adenocarcinoma tissue. (A) Nine clusters were identified by t-SNE analysis. (B) Cluster analysis in each side; sky blue dots indicate the endometrial side (E-side) and red dots are the myometrial infiltration side (M-side). (C) The ratio (%) of macrophages in the E- or M-side of tissues is shown. (D) Relative intensity of CXCL3, CXCL8, and NFKBIA in both sides. *$p < 0.001$ for E-side vs. M-side by the Mann-Whitney U-test. (E) Summary of UCHL1 expression. Relative intensity of UCHL1 is shown, and *$p < 0.001$ for E-side vs. M-side by the Mann-Whitney U-test. (F) Overall survival of Kaplan-Meier estimate was obtained from cBioPortal for CANCER GENOMICS. Blue: control, Red: relatively higher expression group. *$p < 0.001$ for the control vs. high UCHL1 expression.*

hydrolase activity and *UCHIL1* ligase activity may affect the neurodegeneration [17, 18]. In our EA tissue, the relative intensity of *UCHL1* expression was higher on the E-side (**Figure 2E**). The functional role of *UCHL1* in human tumor malignancy is still unresolved, but this gene has been reported to be cancer-related in endometrial cancer patients [19]. Goto et al. demonstrated that activation of *UCHL1* via hypoxia inducible factor-1 (*HIF-1*) is the key regulator for underling mechanism of tumor metastasis, and they expected *UCHL1* is as prognostic marker and treatment target for breast and lung cancers [20].

From the enormous single-cell RNA-sequencing data, the researcher must determine to manage and understand the functional meaning of the cell population. In particular, understanding how the gene is related to overall survival of EA patients in the clinical site is useful. Hence, we used the "cBioPortal For CANCER

GENOMICS" website and chose "Uterine Corpus Endometrial Carcinoma (EC) (TCGA, Provisional)." Subsequently, we set "Genomic profiles" as "mRNA Expression," and chose "mRNA Expression z-Score (microarray)," then input the gene name "*UCHL1*" (http://www.cbioportal.org/). Overall Survival of Kaplan-Meier (K-M) Estimate showed that high *UCHL1* expression in endometrial carcinoma patients significantly decreased survival time (**Figure 2F**). The median months survival in the *UCHL1* high group was 48.75 months. The log-rank $p$ value for K-M analysis for correlation between mRNA expression level and patient survival was $1.965 \times 10^{-4}$. The Overall Survival of K-M Estimate was not calculated from the EA but EC dataset, however EA of the endometrium is the most common type of EC [21]. Therefore, the result indicates that higher expression of *UCHL1* on the E-side somehow affects EA progression, and it supports our hypothesis that cells with HMP are present on the E-side. Whether we chose other data set "Uterine Corpus Endometrial Carcinoma (TCGA, Nature 2013)," the result of Overall Survival of K-M Estimate was also significant ($p = 1.06 \times 10^{-3}$). The median months of disease-free in high *UCHL1* patients was 12.94 months, and it was significantly earlier by the Disease/Progression-free Kaplan-Meier Estimate. However, the significant correlation was not observed if we chose "mRNA Expression z-Scores (RNA Seq V2 RSEM), z-score threshold ± 2.0" ($p = 0.955$). There was other useful database to realize the overall survival of EC patients. We used the "THE HUMAN PROTEIN ATLAS" website and input the gene name "*UCHL1*," then set "PATHOLOGY ATLAS" (http://www.proteinatlas.org/). The prognostic summary highlighted that *UCHL1* was the candidate as the prognostic marker in EC. The 5-year survival in the *UCHL1* high or low group was 66 or 86% respectively, and the $p$ score was $4.1 \times 10^{-5}$ from the total of 541 female patients.

As shown in **Figure 3**, there was significant differences about *UCHL1* expression between each side, and immunostaining of *UCHL1* showed a similar staining

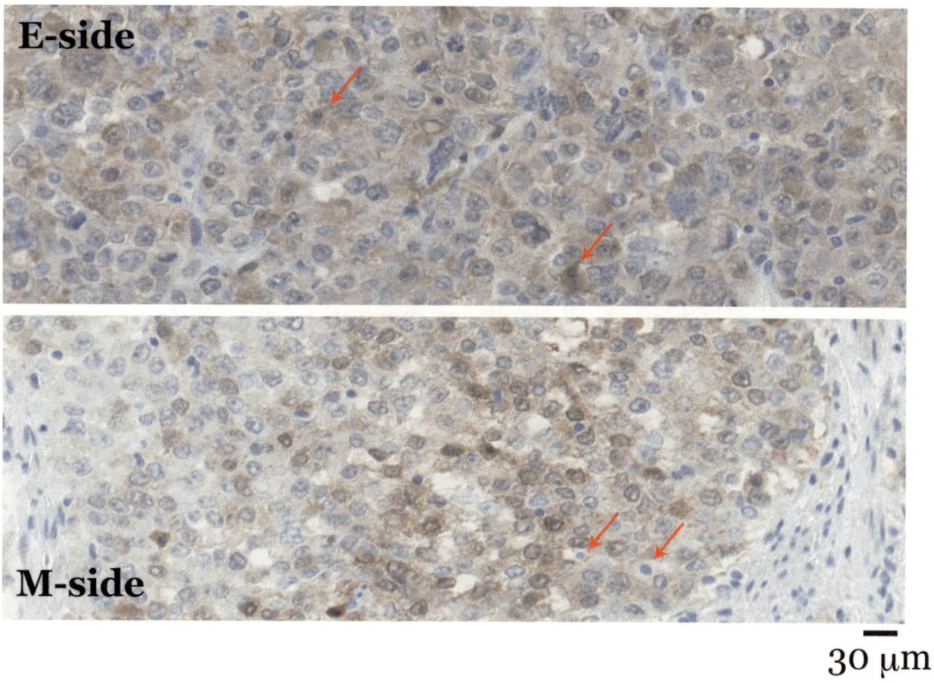


**Figure 3.**
*Immunohistochemistry of UCHL1 in E-side and M-side. Macrophages identified by pathologist are also positively stained. Red allows shows macrophage. The scale bar indicates 30 μm.*

pattern in macrophages as well as cancer cells. Also, *UCHL1* staining in E-side was relatively higher. These data indicate that microenvironment of tumor tissue might affect the gene properties of immune cells, and gene expression pattern might resemble closely to cancer cells.

The high expression of *CXCL3* was not related to the prognosis of EA ($p$ = 0.987) by the CANCER GENOMICS, but *CXCL3* high group significantly improved 5-year overall survival by the PROTEIN ATLAS. At this moment, there was only one patient whose expression of *CXCL8* was high in the CANCER GENOMICS, but 5-year survival of *CXCL8* high or low group in EC patients was 79 or 70% respectively, and there was no significant difference. In contrast, higher expression of *NFKBIA* significantly decreased survival time by "mRNA Expression z-Sore (microarray)" ($p$ = 0.0246), but not "mRNA Expression z-Score (RNA Seq V2 RSEM)" by the CANCER GENOMICS. In contrast, the 5-year overall survival in the PROTEIN ATLAS was not significant. These results indicate that the researcher must use some database to understand how the target genes are related to the prognosis of cancers. Further studies for other HMP-related genes are ongoing in our laboratory.

## 5. Conclusion

Single-cell sequencing is believed to be a powerful tool to answer unknown biological questions, and researchers may have many expectations to find new insights of their hypotheses. Indeed, bulk-based RNA sequencing is averaged across a cell population, but the method to obtain total RNA is relatively simple and easy. Most importantly, we can detect gene expression profiling of the whole tissue. Of course, as mentioned above, the existence of minor cell populations, such as cancer stem-like cells, may not be detected in bulk-based RNA sequencing data. If the researchers knew the biomarkers of targeted cells in small population, the gene can be detected from the bulk-based RNA sequencing data. But it is unknown which cell expresses and how many cells have the targeted gene because of the averaged data by bulk-based RNA sequencing. Thus, it is better to ponder over which method is aimed at the biological question before choosing more difficult and expensive single-cell RNA sequencing.

Current protocols of dispersing single cells in each tissue are not optimized worldwide; therefore, some cells or cell populations may disappear in the course of isolating single cells from tumor tissue. One of the most important procedures for single-cell RNA sequencing is isolation of single cells from tumor tissues. Mechanical and/or enzymatic cell distributed processes followed by fluorescence-activated cell sorting (FACS), magnetic-activated cell sorting (MACS), or density-gradient method are the current standard [22], but the softness or hardness of tissues differs depending on the tumor. Inappropriate single-cell isolation methods are biased; therefore, more detailed studies are needed to optimize isolation of single cells for each tissue.

Nonetheless, single-cell sequencing is a great tool for detecting heterogeneous subpopulations, cell-to-cell communication, and spatial interactions. Moreover, the many gene expression changes by carcinostatic agents can be monitored. To analyze extensively heterogeneous clinical samples, highly sensitive, low cost, quick, and simple technologies to capture mRNA from a single cell are required. Our newly developed single-cell transcriptome analysis, Nx1-seq, can be a useful tool to understand tumor microenvironments with high sensitivity and low cost. This new approach is a simple method, and it can be used to analyze several hundreds to tens of thousands of cells without specialized equipment. Further, it is easy to change the size of the microwell for larger or smaller cells. Furthermore, microwells equipped with bar-code beads in the Nunc™ Lab-Tek™ Chamber slide system can be stored for several months before use. Nx1-seq is a powerful approach for characterizing cellular diversity under physiological and pathological conditions. The combined analysis of t-SNE by Seurat and detailed gene profiling can discover new tumor biomarkers or new target genes for regression of tumor tissues. We continue to develop better Nx1-seq devices to satisfy requests from researchers. It is about continued learning on a daily basis.

## Acknowledgements

The authors would like to thank Y. Kamide, S. Kurokawa, and H. Sekine for technical assistance with the experiments. We also thank A. Tagata for assistance of accounting work. We greatly appreciate Dr. Y. Takamura for supplying PDMS membrane. Prof. T. Torigoe and Dr. Y. Hirohashi gave us the data of UCHL1 immunohistochemistry and constructive comments, thank you. This work is supported by the Japan Agency for Medical Research and Development (AMED). We would like to thank Editage (http://www.editage.jp) for English language editing.

## Conflict of interest

The authors have no conflicts of interest directly relevant to the content of this article.

## Author details

Sadahiro Iwabuchi* and Shinichi Hashimoto
Department of Integrative Medicine for Longevity, Graduate School of Medical Sciences, Kanazawa University, Kanazawa, Ishikawa, Japan

*Address all correspondence to: s_iwabuchi@staff.kanazawa-u.ac.jp

## References

[1] Hashimshony T, Wagner F, Sher N, Yanai I. CEL-seq: Single-cell RNA-Seq by multiplexed linear amplification. Cell Reports. 2012;**2**:666-673. DOI: 10.1016/j.celrep.2012.08.003

[2] Sasagawa Y, Nikaido I, Hayashi T, Danno H, Uno KD, Imai T, et al. Quartz-Seq: A highly reproducible and sensitive single-cell RNA sequencing method, reveals non-genetic gene-expression heterogeneity. Genome Biology. 2013;**14**:R31-47. DOI: 10.1186 gb-2013-14-4-r31

[3] Sasagawa Y, Danno H, Takada H, Ebisawa M, Tanaka K, Hayashi T, et al. Quartz-Seq2: A high-throughput single-cell RNA-sequencing method that effectively uses limited sequence reads. Genome Biology. 2018;**19**:29-52. DOI: 10.1186/s13059-018-1407-3

[4] Picelli S, Faridani OR, Bjroklund AK, Winberg G, Sagasser S, Sandberg R. Full-length RNA-seq from single cells using Smart-seq2. Nature Protocols. 2014;**9**:171-181. DOI: 10.1038/npront.2014.006

[5] Macosko EZ, Basu A, Satija R, Nemesh J, Shekhar K, Goldman M, et al. Highly parallel genome-wide expression profiling of individual cells using nanoliter droplets. Cell. 2015;**161**:1202-1214. DOI: 10.1016/j.cell.2015.05.002

[6] Klein AM, Mazutis L, Akartuna L, Tallapragada N, Veres A, Li V, et al. Droplet barcodeing for single cell transcriptomic applied to embryonic stem cells. Cell. 2015;**161**:1187-1201. DOI: 10.106/j.cell.2015.04.044

[7] Fan X, Zhang X, Wu X, Guo H, Hu Y, Tang F, et al. Single-cell RNA-seq transcriptome analysis of linear and circular RNAs in mouse preimplantation embryos. Genome Biology. 2015;**16**:148-164. DOI: 10.1186/s13059-015-0706-1

[8] Yuan J, Sims PA. An automated microwell platform for large-scale single cell RNA-seq. Scientific Reports. 2016;**6**:33883-33892. DOI: 10.1038/srep33883

[9] Hashimoto S, Tabuchi Y, Yurino H, Hirohashi Y, Deshimaru S, Asano T, et al. Comprehensive single-cell transcriptome analysis reveals heterogeneity in endometrioid adenocarcinoma tissues. Scientific Reports. 2017;**27**:14225-14238. DOI: 10.1038/s41598-017-14676-3

[10] Ziegenhain C, Vieth B, Parekh S, Guillaumet AA, Smets M, Leonhardt H, et al. Comparative anaylsis of single-cell RNA sequencing methods. Molecular Cell. 2017;**65**:631-643. DOI: 10.1016/j.molcel;.2017.01.023

[11] Han X, Wang R, Zhou Y, Fei L, Sun H, Lai S, et al. Mapping the mouse cell atlas by microwell-seq. Cell. 2018;**172**:1091-1107. DOI: 10.1016/j.cell.2018.02.001

[12] Simone P. Single-cell RNA-sequencing: The future of genome biology is now. RNA Biology. 2017;**14**:637-650. DOI: 10.1080/15476286.2016.1201618

[13] Chung W, Eum HH, Lee HO, Lee KM, Lee HB, Lim KT, et al. Single-cell RNA-seq enables comprehensive tumour and immune cell profiling in primary breast cancer. Nature Communications. 2017;**8**:15081. DOI: 10.1038/ncomms15081

[14] DeLaughter DM. The use of the Fluidigm C1 for RNA expression analyses of single cells. Current Protocols in Molecular Biology. 2018;**122**:e55. DOI: 10.1002/cpmb.56

[15] Cazet AS, Hui MN, Elsworth BL, Wu SZ, Roden D, Chan CL, et al. Targeting stromal remodeling and

cancer stem cell plasticity overcomes chemoresistance in triple negative breast cancer. Nature Communications. 2018;**9**:2897-2904. DOI: 10.1038/s41467-018-05220-6

[16] Savas P, Virassamy B, Ye C, Salim A, Mintoff CP, Caramia F, et al. Single-cell profiling of breast cancer T cells reveals a tissue-resident memory subset associated with improved prognosis. Nature Medicine. 2018;**24**:986-993. DOI: 10.1038/s41591-018-0078-7

[17] Liu Y, Fallon L, Lashuel HA, Lansbury PT Jr. The UCH-L1 gene encodes two opposing enzymatic activities that affect alpha-synuclein degradation and Parkinson's disease susceptibility. Cell. 2002;**111**:209-218. DOI: 10.1016/S0092-8674(02)01012-7

[18] Choi J, Al L, Weintraub ST, Rees HD, Gearing M, Chin LS, et al. Oxidative modifications and down-regulation of ubiquitin carboxyl-terminal hydrolase L1 associated with idiopathic Parkinson's and Alzheimer's diseases. The Journal of Biological Chemistry. 2004;**279**:13256-13264. DOI: 10.1074/jbc.M314124200

[19] Nakao K, Hirakawa T, Suwa H, Kogure K, Ikeda S, Yamashita S, et al. High expression of ubiquitin C-terminal hydrolase L1 is associated with poor prognosis in endometrial cancer patiens. International Journal of Gynecological Cancer. 2018;**28**:675-683. DOI: 10.1097/IGC.0000000000001201

[20] Goto Y, Zeng L, Yeom CH, Zhu Y, Morinibu A, Shinomiya K, et al. UCHL1 provides diagnostic and antimetastatic strategies due to its deubiquitinating effect on HIF-1α. Nature Communications. 2015;**6**:6153-6165. DOI: 10.1038/ncomms7153

[21] Morice P, Leary A, Creutzberg C, Abu-Rustum N, Darai E. Endometrial cancer. Lancet. 2016;**387**:1094-1108. DOI: 10.1016/S0140-6736(15)00130-0

[22] Hu P, Zhang W, Xin H, Deng G. Single cell isolation and analysis. Frontiers in Cell and Development Biology. 2016;**4**:116-127. DOI: 10.3389/fcell.2016.00116

Section 3

# Reference Transcriptomes

Chapter 3

# Transcriptome Atlas by Long-Read RNA Sequencing: Contribution to a Reference Transcriptome

*Dong Jin Lee and Chang Pyo Hong*


## Abstract

The recent emergence of long-read transcriptome sequencing has helped improve the overall accuracy of gene prediction compared with that by short-read RNA-Seq. In addition, the technology can offer a more comprehensive view of functional genomics in uncharacterized species with an efficient full-length unigene build and high-precision gene annotation, thus being efficient in developing transcriptome data resources from useful genetic pools. Hence, I will review the applications of long-read RNA isoform sequencing, including the relative merits of the technology, the improvement of the accuracy in gene prediction and gene annotation, and the full-length unigene builds in a new genome; the limitations of the technology will be also discussed. The review will be valuable in collecting data resources for functional genomic studies.


**Keywords:** functional genomics, gene prediction, long-read RNA sequencing, transcriptome

## 1. Introduction

Transcriptomics is the study of transcript catalogs in a cell, tissue, or organism for a given developmental stage or physiological condition [1]. The transcriptome indicates the complete set of transcripts that consists of protein-coding messenger RNA (mRNA) and non-coding RNA (ncRNA), including ribosomal RNA (rRNA), transfer RNA (tRNA), and other ncRNAs [2, 3]. In contrast with the relatively stable genome, various factors such as developmental stage, physiological condition, and external environment influence the changes in the transcriptome. The goals of transcriptomics include the annotation of the transcriptome, and the determination of the functional structure of each gene in the genome and the changes in the expression levels of each gene among different transcriptome samples [1, 4, 5].

Transcriptome analysis depends heavily on the availability of high-throughput tools on account of the complexity of the transcriptome. Thus, RNA sequencing (RNA-Seq) has become an important tool for biological studies. RNA-Seq can quantify gene expression spatially and temporally. Although RNA-Seq has enabled the generation of massive amounts of sequence data due to their high-throughput characteristic, their application of short reads makes them poorly suited for genome and transcriptome assembly, and isoform detection. Single-molecule real-time (SMRT) sequencing, a new method to generate long-read sequences developed by

PacBio platform, provides an alternative approach to overcome these limitations in sequence length and accelerate improving our understanding of the complexity of the transcripts [6].

In general, the read length of Illumina HiSeq platform is about 100–150 bp, which is relatively short compared to that of PacBio platform (around 10 kb). However, Illumina HiSeq platform has the advantage of generating more accurate reads and high-throughput data. On the other hand, even though its accuracy is lower than that of Illumina HiSeq platform, single-molecule real-time (SMRT) sequencing of PacBio platform, a new method of sequence analysis, was developed and applied to elucidate the genomic structures of difficult to sequence organisms [7] because of its long-reads, which results in the improvement of assembly, gene prediction, and annotation. Using this technique, sequences are analyzed from a single strand of DNA without genomic amplification [9]. PCR-free long-read sequencing enables to help to carry out large complex whole-genomes (i.e., hexaploid wheat and maize).

PacBio sequencing captures sequences during the replication process of the target DNA in real-time. The template, also called a SMRTbell, contains a target double-stranded DNA (dsDNA) ligated with hairpin adaptors at both ends, resulting in a closed and single-stranded circular DNA [8]. When the SMRTbell is loaded into a chip called a SMRT cell, diffusion of the SMRTbell into a sequencing unit called a zero-mode wave guide (ZMW) is carried out [10]. In each ZMW, a single polymerase immobilized at the bottom can bind to adaptors of the SMRTbell [11]. Each of the four nucleotides is fluorescent-labeled. As a nucleotide associates with the template in the active site of the polymerase, a light pulse is produced for base detection. A single polymerase read can be generated up to 40 kb, depending on the library size and sequencing time. The closed-circle form of the SMRTbell can make the reaction repeat until the reaction is terminated after the replication of one strand of the target dsDNA or double-stranded complementary DNA by the polymerase. However, the mean length of full transcripts is 1–3 kb in most plant and animal genomes (e.g., 1.6 kb in *Arabidopsis* [12], 1.8 kb in rice [13], 2.3 kb in human [14], and 1.2 kb in mouse [15]); thus, the same transcript can be covered multiple times by the long polymerase read. In this scenario, a few reads (called subreads) can be generated from the polymerase read by trimming adaptor sequences. The consensus sequence of multiple subreads in a single ZMW generates a read of insert (ROI) or a circular consensus sequence (CCS) read with higher accuracy. Hence, a protocol of isoform sequencing (Iso-Seq) for long-read transcriptome sequencing that includes library construction, size selection, sequencing, and data processing was developed by PacBio. Iso-Seq allows the direct sequencing of transcripts up to 10 kb, which is particularly useful for the genomes of uncharacterized species.

However, even though PacBio sequencing has an advantage in terms of read length over next-generation sequencing, the throughput of PacBio sequencing is relatively low. A single SMRT cell contains 150,000 ZMWs, each of which can produce one polymerase read with a mean length of 1o kb. Typically, only 35,000–70,000 reads of the 150,000 ZMW wells on a SMRT cell can be produced successfully because of the failure of anchoring a polymerase and loading more than one DNA molecule in a ZMW. Consequently, the typical throughput of the PacBio RS II system is around 0.5–1 Gb per SMRT cell [16]. Recently, PacBio developed another system called Sequel that produces over seven times the reads, with 1,000,000 ZMWs, and yields around 3.5–7 Gb per SMRT cell [17]. Sequel is appropriate for projects such as *de novo* genome assembly and isoform sequencing of transcriptomes. Another notable problem of PacBio sequencing is the relatively high error rate (around 11–15%) of polymerase reads [18]. Many hybrid sequencing approaches have been attempted to develop a method that has the accuracy of short reads but with the length of PacBio reads [19].

Long-read transcriptome sequencing generates longer and improved transcripts with a high level of assembly completeness and gene annotation. Moreover, it prevents obtaining artifacts such as chimeras, structural errors, incomplete assembly, and base errors [20].

Here, we review the sample preparation, library construction, analytical pipelines, and the result of isoform sequencing (Iso-Seq), as a long-read transcriptome sequencing, in gene prediction and annotation. Furthermore, we will also discuss the relative merits and the limitations of the Iso-Seq technology.

## 2. Merits of long-read transcriptome sequencing

Long-read transcriptome sequencing such as Iso-Seq generates longer and improved transcripts from a species with a high level of assembly completeness and gene annotation, enabling a comprehensive view of the transcriptome. Conventional methods, such as cDNA cloning and EST sequencing, have limitations with relatively low data coverage. Although deep short-read sequencing (i.e., RNA-Seq) provides good sequencing depth and coverage for genome-wide transcriptome analysis, their short-read length generates assembly incompleteness of transcripts, resulting in high error rate in assembly and unreliable gene annotation. Long-read transcriptome sequencing can also provide experimental verification of predicted gene models in a genome, enable the quality of gene structures predicted and also give the potential to reduce missing gene annotation. For example, missing gene annotation may lead to false interpretation such as gene loss and errors in gene expression profiles that map and quantify RNA-seq reads using predicted gene models. Thus, this technology can be helpful to find full-length (FL) transcripts harboring complete open reading frames (ORFs) and uncover novel splice isoforms as well as novel genes. This can result in the improvement of accuracy of gene prediction with an experimental verification and annotations for aiding in studying gene regulation.

## 3. Sample preparation and library construction for isoform sequencing

Iso-Seq with the PacBio platform can generate FL cDNA sequences including the 5′ and 3′-UTRs (untranslated regions), as well as the polyA tails of the transcripts. The whole workflow including the experimental protocol and analytical pipelines is illuminated in **Figure 1** [10].

### 3.1 Isolation of total RNA

The samples can be collected from various tissues (i.e., blood, gill, skin, muscle, liver, spleen, intestine, ovary, testis, kidney, heart, and brain of an animal) [21], or from certain developmental stages (developing rabbit at 21, 49, and 84 days of age) [22]. The high quality of RNA with enough purity and integrity is critical to reduce the amplification cycles required in large-scale PCR and improve the sequencing diversity. RNA extraction is usually done through an easy-spin RNA extraction kit, or RNAiso Pure RNA Isolation kit [20–22]. In general, 2–5 μg of total RNA with an RNA integrity number (RIN) greater than 7 is required.

### 3.2 cDNA synthesis and size partitioning

Isolation of polyA mRNA is required for analyzing the transcripts of protein-coding genes. The Iso-Seq method is flexible and allows different types of RNA

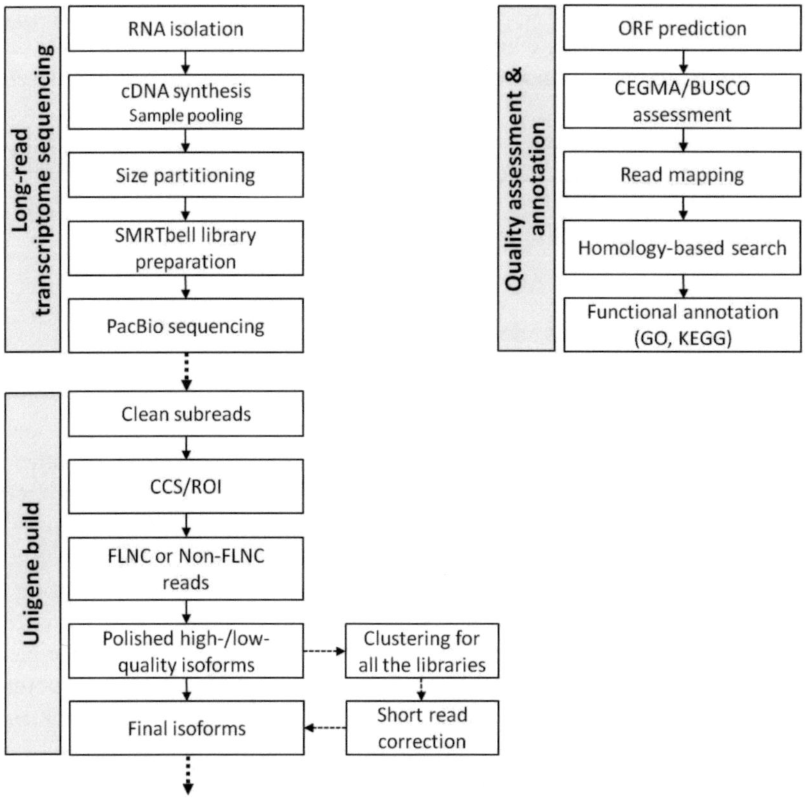


**Figure 1.**
*Schematic workflow of isoform sequencing.*

to be sequenced. Alternatively, mRNAs can be selected by polyA enrichment. The first-strand cDNA is amplified with oligo(dT) to enrich RNAs with a polyA tail, including mRNAs and long noncoding RNAs (lncRNAs) for further analysis.

For parallel analysis of RNA samples derived from various tissues, barcode for each sample with unique sequences is alternatively used. For instance, multiplex sequencing was performed to construct a maize transcriptome library from various tissues [23]. However, barcoding samples is not always desired because sequencing efficiency may be reduced by the barcode sequence.

### 3.3 Size partitioning

Size selection for size partitioning, which is the most commonly used method to avoid over-representation of smaller transcripts in sequencing data, allows for more even representation of cDNA of different size ranges, since smaller fragments may load preferentially on the sequencer. Furthermore, the process of second fractionation is recommended to remove any smaller fractions from the first size selection. To enhance PCR amplification, different sizes of the cDNA libraries including <1, 1–2, 2–3, and 3–6 kb are generally constructed to maximally recover transcript diversity and sequence. However, such size selection may bring about missing small size transcripts less than approximately 1 kb. This problem appears to result from technical limitation by size selection in the construction of mRNA sequencing libraries. This can get solved by combinatorial use with short-read RNA-Seq data that are very effective for transcriptome coverage, especially small size of transcripts.

### 3.4 Library preparation and sequencing

Double-stranded cDNA is not enough for SMRTbell library construction following size selection. PacBio suggests PCR amplification using the KAPA HiFi Enzyme [24] with about 10 cycles. Then, a circularized molecule called a SMRTbell template is transformed from the amplified cDNAs by the SMRTbell Template Prep kit. After the step is completed, the library is ready to be loaded into a SMRT cell and subjected to sequencing on the PacBio platform. There is a compromise between SMRT cell numbers and the sequencing cost. In general, the Iso-Seq protocol recommends 8–50 SMRT cells to retrieve diversity in a tissue.

## 4. Building full-length transcripts in a genome

Error correction of the raw reads is necessary to improve the assembly quality of the FL transcripts. PacBio provides the Iso-Seq analysis software to perform the procedure by iterative clustering for error correction (ICE) and the Quiver algorithm (https://www.pacb.com/applications/rna-sequencing). Then, various analysis approaches can be applied to overcome the limitation of Iso-Seq, improve assembly quality, and evaluate the quality assessment of the unigenes.

The Iso-Seq raw reads are usually called polymerase reads or continuous long reads (CLRs) and have an average length of 10 kb (**Figure 1**). Considering the average length of a transcript is 1–2 kb, the same copies of the inserts are contained in a single polymerase that could be split into several subreads by removing the adaptor sequences by PacBio SMRT link analysis [20]. The circular consensus sequences or ROIs are generated from several subreads. The full-length non-chimeric read (FLNC) is defined not only when the polyA tail signal preceding the 30-primer is present, but also when both 50- and 30-cDNA primers are present. To enhance consensus accuracy and remove the redundancy of FLNC without any additional sequence data, ICE and Quiver can be applied [20]. The Iso-Seq classify tool is used for classifying the ROIs into full-length nonchimeric and non-full-length reads by identifying the 50 and 30 adapters used in library preparation. Then, the Iso-Seq cluster tool is used for clustering all the full-length reads, and the consensus sequences produced by the cluster tool are polished using the non-full-length reads through the Quiver algorithm [25]. Additionally, the CD-HIT program [26] is likely to be helpful to cluster the high and low quiver consensus isoforms from ROIs with high sequence identity threshold (i.e. 0.98–0.99) [20, 21].

Iso-Seq reads present a disadvantage with the high frequency of errors of nucleotide indels and mismatches. Thus, the procedure of correcting InDels and mismatches is performed via alignment with reference genomes [27]. To overcome this, a viable alternative approach is to integrate short reads with long reads via hybrid sequencing. For instance, RNA samples prepared from the same samples are sequenced by both PacBio and Illumina HiSeq. The short reads from the Illumina HiSeq are applied to correct the transcript isoforms using LoRDEC tool v0.6 [28]. Then, the corrected isoform sequences are aligned against a reference genome by GMAP aligner [29]. The following analyses are recommended to exclude the sequences with multiple and chimeric alignments. To assess quality of the unigenes, some software such as CEGMA [30] and BUSCO [31] can be applied [20, 21, 32, 33]. The percentages of the transcripts that fully and partially aligned to the conserved proteins are calculated.

FL or longer transcriptome data have been mostly published from large complex or uncharacterized genomes of plant species (**Table 1**). Although deep short-read transcriptome sequencing (i.e., RNA-Seq) have accumulated over recent year, they are likely to generate low-quality transcripts with a small portion of FL transcripts, prohibiting accurate transcript reconstruction and leading incorrect annotation.

| Species | No. of transcripts | Mean length (bp) | Discovery | | | | | Reference |
|---|---|---|---|---|---|---|---|---|
| | | | Identification of novel gene isoforms | Isoform annotation | Alternative splicing events | Gene prediction | Other | |
| *Panax ginseng* | 135,317 | 3178 | Y | Y | Y | — | — | [20] |
| *Triticum aestivum* | 91,881 | 2388 | Y | Y | — | — | — | [45] |
| *Zea mays* B73 | 111,151 | 3372 | Y | Y | Y | Y | Fusion transcripts | [23] |
| *Sorghum bicolor* | 27,860 | 1042 (full-length ROI) | Y | Y | Y | Y | — | [27] |
| *Trifolium pratense* | 206,465 | 2789 | Y | Y | Y | — | — | [34] |
| *Zea mays* W64A | 166,693 | 2715 | Y | Y | Y | — | Fusion transcripts | [35] |
| *Allium sativum* | 36,321 | 1500 | Y | Y | — | — | Association study | [36] |
| *Populus* (*P. deltoides* × *P. euramericana* cv. 'Nanlin895') | 87,150 | 2417 | Y | Y | Y | — | Fusion transcripts | [37] |
| *Coffea arabica* | 95,995 | 3236 | Y | Y | Y | Y | — | [38] |

**Table 1.**
*Transcriptomics studies in plants by isoform sequencing.*

vUnlike RNA-Seq data, Iso-Seq data, which are derived from various tissues as many as possible, harbor a large portion of unique FL transcripts. For example, Wang et al. [23] reported that maize yielded 111,151 non-redundant FL transcript isoforms, corresponding to approximately 26,946 genes. In addition, genome coverage of Iso-Seq data is achieved near-saturation. Ultimately, cost-effective long-read transcriptome sequencing can be the gold standard for transcript completeness, characterization of transcriptome, and draft genome annotation. To identify trait-associated transcripts in species for which a reference genome is lacking (i.e., garlic), this approach was used as a reference sequence for scoring the variation in both SNP and expression level in the population [36], reporting the characterization of transcripts (lncRNAs) associated with garlic clove shape traits.

## 5. Improvement of the efficiency of functional gene prediction and annotation

Completeness of assembled transcripts is closely related to the efficiency of functional gene prediction or annotation, especially in the absence of reference genome information. Because of such advantage, Iso-Seq has been applied in a variety of species [20–22, 32, 33]. In addition, optimized training and prediction settings on the basis of short- and long-read transcriptome data in gene prediction results in increased their sensitivity and precision [39]. In particular, the method is helpful for obtaining comprehensive gene sets for newly sequenced genomes of non-model eukaryotes [39].

To identify the protein coding potential of transcripts, Transdecoder (https://transdecoder.github.io) is generally applied [20, 21, 32, 40]. For example, even though the number of transcripts using Iso-Seq is much smaller than those *de novo* assembled in previous RNA-seq studies, the transcripts from Iso-Seq show high efficiency in recovering full-length transcripts. ESTScan [41], in addition to Transdecoder, is used to predict coding DNA sequences (CDSs) unless isoforms are annotated in the databases. For example, in the study of *Halogeton glomeratus* [42], the CDS prediction ratio of transcripts using Iso-Seq (95.09%) is much higher than that of transcripts using Illumina RNA-Seq data (66.86%).

For functional annotation, isoform sequences are used as queries for sequence homology searches in Blast, Blast2GO [43], and InterProScan5 [44] to identify functional annotation terms from the nonredundant protein (NR), non-redundant nucleotide (NT), Gene Ontology (GO), Clusters of Orthologous Groups (COG), Kyoto Encyclopedia of Genes and Genomes (KEGG), SwissProt, and Interpro databases. For example, when the RNA-Seq data of *H. glomeratus* were re-annotated with Iso-Seq transcriptome data, the length distribution, functional annotation, and coding sequence quantity of the Iso-Seq transcripts were significantly improved [42]. In particular, with respect to the species distribution of the annotation from the NR database, 98.31% of the annotated isoforms showed the highest similarity to sequences from the three most prevalent species. In addition, Illumina RNA-Seq data were highly mapped to the Iso-Seq transcripts (unigenes). This suggests that long-read, full-length or partial-unigene data with high-quality assemblies are invaluable resources as transcriptomic references in a genome and can be used for comparative analyses in closely related medicinal plants.

## 6. Conclusion

Transcriptome data generated by Iso-Seq generate longer and improved unigenes with a high level of assembly completeness and gene annotation, enabling a comprehensive view of the transcriptome. In particular, compared with conventional methods, long-read transcriptome sequencing seems to improve misassembly rate and unreliable gene annotation, thus enabling to elucidate the function of genes associated with traits of interest as well as novel transcripts. A hybrid approach that combines isoform sequencing with full-length transcripts and RNA-Seq capable of fixing sequence error and quantifying gene expression is the optimal solution to study transcriptomes for improving completeness of transcripts, data coverage, and gene annotation.

## Acknowledgements

This work was supported by grants from the National Agricultural Genome Center (project No. PJ01349002), Rural Development Administration, Republic of Korea.

## Conflict of interest

The author declares no conflict of interest to disclose.

## Author details

Dong Jin Lee and Chang Pyo Hong*
Theragen Etex Bio Institute, Suwon, Republic of Korea

*Address all correspondence to: changpyo.hong@theragenetex.com

## References

[1] Tang F et al. mRNA-Seq whole-transcriptome analysis of a single cell. Nature Methods. 2009;**6**:377-382. DOI: 10.1038/nmeth.1315

[2] Lindberg J, Lundeberg J. The plasticity of the mammalian transcriptome. Genomics. 2010;**95**:1-6. DOI: 10.1016/j.ygeno.2009.08.010

[3] Okazaki Y et al. Analysis of the mouse transcriptome based on functional annotation of 60,770 full-length cDNAs. Nature. 2002;**420**:563-573. DOI: 10.1038/nature01266

[4] Costa V, Angelini C, De Feis I, Ciccodicola A. Uncovering the complexity of transcriptomes with RNA-Seq. Journal of Biomedicine & Biotechnology. 2010:19. DOI: 10.1155/2010/853916 Article ID 853916

[5] Ruan Y, Le Ber P, Ng HH, Liu ET. Interrogating the transcriptome. Trends in Biotechnology. 2004;**22**(1):23-30. DOI: 10.1016/j.tibtech.2003.11.002

[6] Rhoads A, Au KF. PacBio sequencing and its applications. Genomics, Proteomics & Bioinformatics. 2015;**13**:278-289. DOI: 10.1016/j.gpb.2015.08.002

[7] Sharon D, Tilgner H, Grubert F, Snyder M. A single-molecule long-read survey of the human transcriptome. Nature Biotechnology. 2013;**31**:1009-1014

[8] Travers KJ et al. A flexible and efficient template format for circular consensus sequencing and SNP detection. Nucleic Acids Research. 2010;**38**(15):e159. DOI: 10.1093/nar/gkq543

[9] Roberts RJ, Carneiro MO, Schatz MC. The advantages of SMRT sequencing. Genome Biology. 2013;**14**:405

[10] Gonzalez-Garay ML. Introduction to isoform sequencing using Pacific Biosciences technology (Iso-Seq). Vol. 9. Dordrecht, The Netherlands: Springer; 2015. pp. 141-160

[11] Eid J, Fehr A, Gray J, Luong K, Lyle J, Otto G, et al. Real-time DNA sequencing from single polymerase molecules. Science. 2009;**323**:133-138. DOI: 10.1126/science.1162986

[12] Swarbreck D et al. The Arabidopsis Information Resource (TAIR): Gene structure and function annotation. Nucleic Acids Research. 2008;**36**(Database issue):D1009-D1014. DOI: 10.1093/nar/gkm965

[13] Ouyang S et al. The TIGR Rice Genome Annotation Resource: Improvements and new features. Nucleic Acids Research. 2007;**35**(Database issue):D883-D887. DOI: 10.1093/nar/gkl976

[14] Ota T et al. Complete sequencing and characterization of 21,243 full-length human cDNAs. Nature Genetics. 2004;**36**(1):40-45. DOI: 10.1038/ng1285

[15] Kawai J et al. Functional annotation of a full-length mouse cDNA collection. Nature. 2001;**409**(6821):685-690. DOI: 10.1038/35055500

[16] PacBio RS II System. Available online: http://dnatech.genomecenter.ucdavis.edu/pacbio-library-prepsequencing [Accessed: 1 November 2017]

[17] PacBio Sequel System. Available online: http://www.pacb.com/products-and-services/pacbio-systems/sequel [Accessed: 12 July 2017]

[18] Korlach J. Understanding accuracy in SMRT® Sequencing. Available online: https://www.pacb.com/wp-content/uploads/2015/09/Perspective_UnderstandingAccuracySMRTSequencing.pdf

[19] Koren S et al. Hybrid error correction and de novo assembly of single-molecule sequencing reads. Nature Biotechnology. 2012;**30**:693-700. DOI: 10.1038/nbt.2280

[20] Jo IH, Lee J, Hong CE, Lee DJ, et al. Isoform sequencing provides a more comprehensive view of the *Panax ginseng* transcriptome. Genes. 2017;**8**:228. DOI: 10.3390/genes8090228

[21] Yi S, Zhou X, Li J, Zhang M, Luo S. Full-length transcriptome of *Misgurnus anguillicaudatus* provides insights into evolution of genus *Misgurnus*. Scientific Reports. 2018;**8**(1):11699. DOI: 10.1038/s41598-018-29991-6

[22] Chen SY, Deng F, Jia X, Li C, Lai SJ. A transcriptome atlas of rabbit revealed by PacBio single-molecule long-read sequencing. Scientific Reports. 2017;**7**(1):7648. DOI: 10.1038/s41598-017-08138-z

[23] Wang B et al. Unveiling the complexity of the maize transcriptome by single-molecule long-read sequencing. Nature Communications. 2016;**7**(11708). DOI: 10.1038/ncomms11708

[24] PacBio SMRTbell library construction. Available online: http://www.pacb.com/products-and-services/analytical-software/devnet [Accessed: 10 May 2017]

[25] Gordon SP et al. Widespread polycistronic transcripts in fungi revealed by single-molecule mRNA sequencing. PLoS One. 2015;**10**(7):e0132628. DOI: 10.1371/journal.pone.0132628

[26] Huang Y, Niu B, Gao Y, Fu L, Li W. CD-HIT Suite: A web server for clustering and comparing biological sequences. Bioinformatics. 2010;**26**(5):680-682. DOI: 10.1093/bioinformatics/btq003

[27] Abdel-Ghany SE et al. A survey of the sorghum transcriptome using single-molecule long reads. Nature Communications. 2016;**7**:11706. DOI: 10.1038/ncomms11706

[28] Salmela L, Rivals E. LoRDEC: Accurate and efficient long read error correction. Bioinformatics. 2014;**30**(24):3506-3514. DOI: 10.1093/bioinformatics/btu538

[29] Wu TD, Watanabe CK. GMAP: A genomic mapping and alignment program for mRNA and EST sequences. Bioinformatics. 2005;**21**(9):1859-1875. DOI: 10.1093/bioinformatics/bti310

[30] Parra G, Bradnam K, Korf I. CEGMA: A pipeline to accurately annotate core genes in eukaryotic genomes. Bioinformatics. 2007;**23**(9):1061-1067. DOI: 10.1093/bioinformatics/btm071

[31] Simão FA, Waterhouse RM, Ioannidis P, Kriventseva EV, Zdobnov EM. BUSCO: Assessing genome assembly and annotation completeness with single-copy orthologs. Bioinformatics. 2015;**31**(19):3210-3212. DOI: 10.1093/bioinformatics/btv351

[32] Zeng D et al. Single-molecule long-read sequencing facilitates shrimp transcriptome research. Scientific Reports. 2018;**8**(1):16920. DOI: 10.1038/s41598-018-35066-3

[33] Pootakham W et al. Development of a novel reference transcriptome for scleractinian coral *Porites lutea* using single-molecule long-read isoform sequencing (Iso-Seq). Frontiers in Marine Science. 2018;**5**(122). DOI: 10.3389/fmars.2018.00122

[34] Chao Y, Yuan J, Li S, Jia S, Han L, Xu L. Analysis of transcripts and splice isoforms in red clover (*Trifolium pratense* L.) by single-molecule long-read sequencing. BMC Plant Biology. 2018;**18**(1):300. DOI: 10.1186/s12870-018-1534-8

[35] Zhou Y, Zhao Z, Zhang Z, Fu M, Wu Y, Wang W. Isoform sequencing provides insight into natural genetic diversity in maize. Plant Biotechnology Journal [Epub ahead of print. 2018. DOI: 10.1111/pbi.13063

[36] Chen X, Liu X, Zhu S, Tang S, Mei S, Chen J, et al. Transcriptome-referenced association study of clove shape traits in garlic. DNA Research. 2018;**25**(6):587-596. DOI: 10.1093/dnares/dsy027

[37] Chao Q, Gao ZF, Zhang D, Zhao BG, Dong FQ, Fu CX, et al. The developmental dynamics of the Populus stem transcriptome. Plant Biotechnology Journal. 2019;**17**(1):206-219. DOI: 10.1111/pbi.12958

[38] Cheng B, Furtado A, Henry RJ. Long-read sequencing of the coffee bean transcriptome reveals the diversity of full-length transcripts. Gigascience. 2017;**6**(11):1-13. DOI: 10.1093/gigascience/gix086

[39] Minoche AE, Dohm JC, Schneider J, Holtgräwe D, Viehöver P, Montfort M, et al. Exploiting single-molecule transcript sequencing for eukaryotic gene prediction. Genome Biology. 2015;**16**(184). DOI: 10.1186/s13059-015-0729-7

[40] Haas BJ, Papanicolaou A, et al. De novo transcript sequence reconstruction from RNA-seq using the Trinity platform for reference generation and analysis. Nature Protocols. 2013;**8**(8):1494-1512. DOI: 10.1038/nprot.2013.084

[41] Iseli C, Jongeneel CV, Bucher P. ESTScan: A program for detecting, evaluating, and reconstructing potential coding regions in EST sequences. Proceedings. International Conference on Intelligent Systems for Molecular Biology. 1999:138-148

[42] Wang J et al. Single-molecule long-read transcriptome dataset of halophyte *Halogeton glomeratus*. Frontiers in Genetics. 2017;**8**(197). DOI: 10.3389/fgene.2017.00197

[43] Conesa A, Götz S, García-Gómez JM, Terol J, Talón M, Robles M. Blast2GO: A universal tool for annotation, visualization and analysis in functional genomics research. Bioinformatics. 2005;**21**(18):3674-3676. DOI: 10.1093/bioinformatics/bti610

[44] Quevillon E, Silventoinen V, Pillai S, Harte N, Mulder N, Apweiler R, et al. InterProScan: Protein domains identifier. Nucleic Acids Research. 2005;**33**(Web Server issue):W116-W120. DOI: 10.1093/nar/gki4

[45] Dong L et al. Single-molecule realtime transcript sequencing facilitates common wheat genome annotation and grain transcriptome research. BMC Genomics. 2015;**16**(1039). DOI: 10.1186/s12864-015-2257-y

Section 4

# Transcriptome Analysis in Plants

Chapter 4

# Plant Comparative Transcriptomics Reveals Functional Mechanisms and Gene Regulatory Networks Involved in Anther Development and Male Sterility

*Xiangyuan Wan and Ziwen Li*

## Abstract

Gene transcription and transcriptional regulation are crucial biological processes in all cellular life. Through the next-generation sequencing (NGS) technology, transcriptome data from different tissues and developmental stages can be easily obtained, which provides us a powerful tool to reveal the transcriptional landscape of investigated tissue(s) at special developmental stage(s). Anther development is an important process not only for sexual plant reproduction but also for genic male sterility (GMS) used in agriculture production. Plant comparative transcriptomics has been widely used to uncover molecular mechanism of GMS. Here, we focused on researches of anther developmental process and plant GMS genes by using comparative transcriptomics method. In detail, the contents include the following: (1) we described the commonly used flowchart in comparative transcriptomics; (2) we summarized the comparative strategies used to analyze transcriptome data; (3) we presented a case study on a maize GMS gene, *ZmMs33*; (4) we described the methods and results previously reported on gene co-expression and gene regulatory networks; (5) we presented the workflow of a case study on gene regulatory network reconstruction. The further development of comparative transcriptomics will provide us more powerful theoretical and application tools to investigate molecular mechanism underlying anther development and plant male sterility.

**Keywords:** plant comparative transcriptomics, gene regulatory network, anther development, genic male sterility, molecular mechanism

## 1. Introduction

Gene transcription is an important biological process by which genetic information stored within DNA molecules is transmitted to RNA molecules according to the "genetic central dogma" in molecular biology [1]. After completion of the human genome project, the researchers began to reveal the transcriptional landscape of all genes in a genome to further investigate the functional mechanisms underlying phenotypic variations at a genome-wide transcriptional level. Therefore, biological studies on high-throughput omics data run from the genomic level into the transcriptomic level. Transcriptome data includes biological information of gene transcriptional activities in a certain cell, a tissue, or an individual (a population of cells) and even in a pool of samples under a certain developmental stage, an environmental condition, or an experimental treatment. Compared with other omics data (e.g., data of genome, epigenome, proteome, metabolome, or phenome), the primary characteristic of transcriptome data is that it includes temporal–spatial bioinformation affected by diverse developmental stages, tissue types, and internal/external environment events. Therefore, transcriptome data is more complex than genome data.

Transcriptomic studies usually focus on the transcriptional content and gene regulations in a genome. Gene expression microarray (GEM) is an early developed but still-utilized biotechnology by which the genome-wide transcription information can be obtained for genome-sequenced or transcriptional loci available species. In 1995, Schena et al. monitored expression levels of 48 genes by GEM in *Arabidopsis thaliana* [2], and then GEM was gradually and widely used for the estimation of gene expression levels. Until 2013, the amount of transcripts monitored by one microarray had been reached to more than 285,000 in human transcriptomics studies (the human transcriptome array). GEM is a hybrid-based method, while the sequencing-based method has been developed much faster and became one of the most commonly used biotechnologies in scientific studies and applications related to disease diagnosis [3]. Serial analysis of gene expression (SAGE) proposed by Velculescu et al. [4] and massively parallel signature sequencing (MPSS) reported by Brenner et al. [5] are two earlier developed sequencing-based methods to estimate the transcription information at a genome level. Nowadays, the majority of transcriptome data are generated by the NGS-based RNA sequencing (RNA-seq). RNA-seq technology combining with the following developed comparative transcriptomics analysis flowchart that is mainly based on digital gene expression profile (DGEP) is a commonly used research strategy in biological studies at molecular and genomic levels.

Anther is an important organ in sexual plant reproduction. Anther development is a dynamic process from the identity of the stamen to the production of mature pollen grains. During this period, two-thirds of protein-coding genes are transcribed, and more than 6% of them are anther specific (a reanalyzed result based on [6]). Thus, the anther transcriptome is specific and complex compared with transcriptomes of other plant organs. Plant comparative transcriptomics is an effective strategy used to investigate the molecular mechanism underlying anther developmental process. The comparative method based on anther transcriptomes can be performed between different genotypes, different developmental stages, different types of anther cells, and different biotic or abiotic treatments and even between different plant species. Consequently, differentially expressed genes (DEGs) are identified from above comparisons. Based on the comparison results, functionally important coding genes and noncoding transcripts including long noncoding RNAs (lncRNAs), microRNAs (miRNAs), and other small RNAs could be uncovered. However, the goal of plant comparative transcriptomics is not only to identify DEGs but also to reconstruct gene regulatory relationships of the upstream regulators and the downstream regulated targets of the investigated genes. In this review, based on anther transcriptomes, we first summarized the research workflow commonly used in the experimental design and data analyses in plant transcriptomics studies, and then we described several types of comparison strategies in comparative transcriptomics using anther transcriptome data as the analyzed example. In the following section, we generally discussed gene regulatory and co-expression networks used to investigate the molecular foundation of developing anther in a network-based perspective. Additionally, we described two case studies in our laboratory to explain the detailed analysis processes and applications of comparative transcriptomics in plant GMS gene studies.

## 2. Comparative analysis using transcriptome data

In comparative transcriptomics, the commonly used pipeline to identify potential functional genes and to reveal the gene functions, as well as to investigate the regulatory relationships between these genes, includes five aspects. They are data preparation, DGEP analysis, DEG analysis, gene set enrichment (GSE) analysis, and gene regulatory network (GRN) analysis, respectively (**Figure 1**). These five aspects are closely connected in the whole pipeline, and the corresponding analyses mainly depend on data management skills in bioinformatics.

The basic application of comparative transcriptomics is to obtain a transcriptional landscape of the investigated biological sample. It is composed of not only the estimated transcription levels of annotated transcribed loci along the genomes (the known genomic loci with reported or predicted transcription abilities) but also the identification of novel transcribed loci (the stably transcribed loci not annotated or identified in previous studies). More importantly, in current biological studies, transcribed loci identified by researchers include not only the protein-coding genes but also lncRNAs and other noncoding RNAs. Both GEM and RNA-seq technologies can be used to uncover the genome-wide profiles of transcription levels of annotated genes. However, the identification of novel transcribed loci can be only effectively performed by RNA-seq method and the following DGEP analysis. This is one reason why RNA-seq is more commonly used in transcriptomics studies. Moreover, GEM method depends on hybridization probes that are designed based on known whole genome sequence or an appreciable set of sequenced transcripts

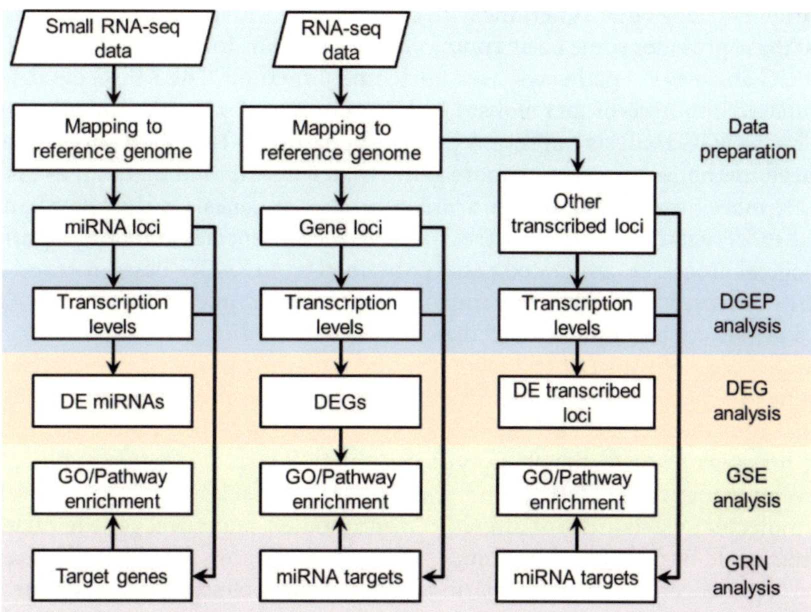


**Figure 1.**
*A flowchart of comparative transcriptomics analysis.*

(e.g., expressed sequence tags) of the investigated species, which restrict its application on some species without whole genome information or sequence resource. On the contrary, the sequencing-based method of RNA-seq can be applicable for species without sequenced genomes. This is another reason for the popularity of RNA-seq. In genome available species, RNA-seq data should be firstly mapped to the reference genome (**Figure 1**).

A gene with its transcription levels significantly different between two groups of samples is defined as a DEG under a certain comparison condition (**Figure 1**). It is notable that the concept of DEG specially represents the expression changes of protein-coding genes at the earlier stages of expression data analysis. However, along with the rapid development of molecular biology and the deeper understanding on the functional element on the genome, the concept of DEG has been expanded to noncoding transcripts, for example, the differentially expressed (DE) miRNA and the DE lncRNA. Furthermore, if both coding and noncoding transcripts are considered in the comparative analysis of transcriptome data, transcriptional alterations between control and treated samples should be defined as DE transcribed loci or DE loci. Thus, DE loci is a broad concept used to describe transcriptional alterations of genetic element. There are several strategies for comparing transcriptomes from different research subjects to identify DE loci (described in Section 3, "Plant comparative transcriptomics in anther").

Identified DEG set or DE loci should be appropriately annotated with functional descriptions to determine which biological process or pathway these DEGs are involved in. In comparative transcriptomics, this step is a critical bridge linking transcriptional changes to gene functions and even gene regulation networks. Two commonly utilized methods to annotate DEGs consist of the Gene Ontology (GO) and the Kyoto Encyclopedia of Genes and Genomes (KEGG) pathway gene enrichment analyses. Both of them belong to GSE analysis (**Figure 1**). The GO database includes tens of thousands of GO terms, and each GO term contains several genes with the same biological function. Each gene has three functional aspects, including molecular function (the molecular activities of gene products), cellular component (the cellular locations of functional gene products), and biological process (the gene products' molecular functions with biological process). GSE analysis based on GO database provides some basic functional descriptions for the investigated DEG set. KEGG analysis is a pathway-based enrichment method. The KEGG database has accumulated hundreds of metabolism pathways in plants, animals, and other species. Thus, KEGG analysis can reveal significant pathways the DEGs participated in. GO-based methods can annotate more genes than KEGG-based method, as the GO terms are more flexible and include a larger number of genes. On the other hand, because most metabolic pathways are conserved across species and more significant in biological processes, annotated results obtained from KEGG-based method may be more conserved and stable. In comparative transcriptomics, GO- and KEGG-based analyses are together utilized in gene function studies.

The locations of transcribed loci on the genome, their transcription levels, and the changed expression can be identified through comparative transcriptomics analysis. The detected DEG set represents a functional gene set related to the function of investigated gene, the phenotype variation, the stress resistance ability, or the development process. Furthermore, gene regulation relationships are the underlining molecular mechanism of altered transcriptomes, and novel gene regulatory networks could be uncovered by comparative transcriptomics analysis (**Figure 1**). Several types of gene regulatory relationships and the reconstructions of gene regulatory networks based on plant comparative transcriptomics are described and discussed in Section 5 ("Gene co-expression and regulatory networks reconstructed by comparative transcriptomics method").

## 3. Plant comparative transcriptomics in anther

One of the major subjects of modern molecular biology is to uncover the functions of genes in the genome and reveal the molecular mechanism of phenotypic variation. Gene transcription levels and their changes in different conditions are important information that can reflect the functions and transcriptional regulation relationships of investigated genes. How to estimate the transcription levels of genes and how to obtain the transcriptional landscape of a genome are two major subjects in biological studies on gene expression. DGEP and DEG analyses are powerful tools to solve these questions. In DEG analysis, according to the scientific or application questions, the comparison strategies between investigated biological samples are classified into six types including (1) different genotypes, (2) different developmental stages, (3) different tissues, (4) different cell types, (5) different treatments, and (6) different species (**Figure 2**). Here, as we mainly focus on comparative transcriptomics analysis on the developmental anther tissues and the interspecies analysis on anther transcriptome data being rare, the third and sixth types will not be discussed.

### 3.1 Different genotypes

There are two types of genotype-based transcriptome data between wild type (WT) and mutant lines in GMS studies, which are based on whether the causal mutation is known or not (**Table 1**). For transcriptomes of male sterility (MS) lines with known causal mutations, the comparison of transcriptomes between WT and MS lines will identify many DEGs associated with the function loss or expression change of the investigated mutation locus. If the causal mutation has not been identified from the MS line, comparative transcriptomics analyses will provide the researchers important results related to the unsettled genetic difference, such as how many genes are changed in expression levels in the MS lines and what the functions of these genes are, even though the causal mutation candidates can be inferred from these genes if the researchers have primary mapping results.

### 3.2 Different developmental stages

The phenotypic differences among tissues and organs (e.g., root, leaf, and flower in plant) due to their differences of transcriptome landscape are well known.

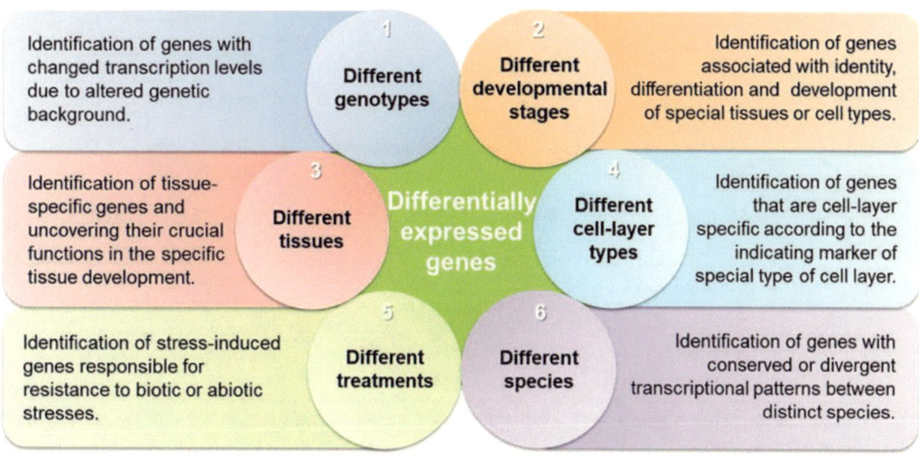


**Figure 2.**
*Comparative transcriptomics strategies.*

| Plants | MS gene or MS line | Method | Tissue | Data source[a] | Reference |
|---|---|---|---|---|---|
| *Arabidopsis thaliana* | *ROXY1* and *ROXY2* | Microarray | Young inflorescences | SD | [7] |
| | *AMS* | Microarray | Anthers | GSE18225 | [8] |
| | *AMS* | Microarray | Anthers | SD | [9] |
| | *AMS* | Microarray | Floral buds | SD | [10] |
| | *EMS1* | Microarray | Anthers | SD | [9] |
| | *EMS1* | Microarray | Anthers | SD | [11] |
| | *Ms1* | Microarray | Young closed buds | SD | [12] |
| | *Ms1* | Microarray | Floral buds | GSE8864 | [13] |
| | *ICE1* | RNA-seq | Anthers | GSE107260 | [14] |
| | *DYT1* | Microarray | Anthers | GSE18225 | [8] |
| | *CDM1* | Microarray | Young floral buds | GSE55799 | [15] |
| | *TEK* | Microarray | Closed floral buds | GSE56497 | [16] |
| | *bHLH010, bHLH08, bHLH091* | RNA-seq | Anthers | SRS838170, SRS838173 | [17] |
| *Oryza sativa* | *PTC1* | Microarray | Anthers | SD | [18] |
| | *UDT1* | Microarray | Anthers | GSE2619 | [19] |
| | *OsGAMYB* | Microarray | Anthers | SD | [20] |
| | *TDR* | Microarray | Spikelets | SD | [21] |
| | *MADS3* | Microarray | Anthers | SD | [22] |
| *Zea mays* | *Ms23* | RNA-seq | Anthers | GSE90849 | [23] |
| | *Ms32* | Microarray | Anthers | GSE90968 | [23] |
| | *MAC1* | Microarray | Anthers | SD | [24] |
| *Triticum aestivum* | *TaMs1* | RNA-seq | Anthers | SRP113349 | [25] |
| | *TaMs2* | RNA-seq | Anthers | SRP092366 | [26] |
| *Solanum lycopersicum* | *ms1035* | RNA-seq | Floral buds | SD | [27] |
| | MS line *7B-1* | RNA-seq | Anthers | GSE85859 | [28] |
| *Brassica napus* | MS line *WSLA* | RNA-seq | Young flower buds | SRR2192464, SRR2192489 | [29] |
| | MS line *SP2S* | RNA-seq | Young flower buds | GSE69638 | [30] |
| | MS line *TE5A* | RNA-seq | Young flower buds | SRP068170 | [31] |
| *Citrullus lanatus* | MS line *DAH3615-MS* | RNA-seq | Floral buds and flowers | GSE69073 | [32] |

[a]*"SD" indicates the raw data is unavailable, while the up- and downregulated genes are listed in the supplemental data (SD) in references cited.*

**Table 1.**
*Published studies on anther transcriptome data between WT and MS lines.*

Furthermore, it is a developmental process for most types of plant organs from the organ identity (e.g., meristematic cells) to the final mature organ. Thus, how to reveal the dynamic changes of gene transcription levels and how to explain the morphological alterations regulated by gene expression changes are important tasks in plant comparative transcriptomics studies.

Meiosis is an important step in gametophyte generation process and sexual plant reproduction. Morphologic changes during cell meiosis process have been well described by cellular level investigations, while the molecular level alterations and their corresponding gene regulatory networks are not well understood. Plant transcriptomes are a powerful dataset to estimate the gene expression changes and infer the regulatory roles of key genes. Based on GEM technology, Ma et al. investigated maize anther transcriptomes during seven developmental stages and found that transcriptomes during meiosis stages exhibited the lowest complexity [33]. Hollender et al. surveyed the gene transcription profiles of anther of woodland strawberry (*Fragaria vesca*) from developmental stages 7–12 and identified numerous F-Box genes induced in transcription levels at meiosis stage [34]. Besides, tapetum is the inner cell layer of anther with important functions in anther development and gametocyte maturation. The generation, development, and degradation of tapetum are fine regulated during the anther development, while the regulatory framework and the details are far from complete. Yue et al. identified 243 DEG and 108 stage-specific genes during four anther developmental stages in *Hamelia patens* [35]. Chen et al. investigated the expression of genes involving in tapetum development of male floral bud during eight developmental stages in *Populus tomentosa* [36]. Thus, anther transcriptome data during different developmental stages provide valuable data sources for anther development studies. By the combination of comparative transcriptomics and bioinformatics analyses, more key functional genes and the underlying regulatory mechanisms for anther development will be further revealed.

### 3.3 Different types of anther cells

The cytological structure of anther consists of four cell layers, including the epidermis, endothecium, middle layer, and tapetum, and the archesporial cells are directly surrounded by the tapetum. Thus, the transcriptome data of a whole anther tissue is a mixed gene expression data from diverse cell types with different functions in the anther development process. It is necessary to obtain transcriptional dynamics from different cell layers separately to investigate anther development and the underlying molecular mechanism at a cell type-specific level. Several studies have identified cell layer-specifically expressed genes (e.g., tapetum cells or microgametes). Ma et al. identified 104 MS-related and non-pollen expressed genes most specifically expressed in tapetum by comparative transcriptomics analysis on four diverse MS lines in *Brassica oleracea* [37]. The other way to obtain cell layer-specific transcriptome in anther is firstly separating the investigated cell layer by laser capture microdissection (LCM) technology and then performing RNA-seq or GEM experiment on the separated samples. This strategy has been successfully used in rice, maize, and woodland strawberry to identify the tapetum- or microgamete-specifically expressed genes and their expression dynamics [34, 38, 39]. A recent published research has investigated maize male meiosis using single-cell RNA sequencing (scRNA-seq) technology on pre-meiotic and meiotic cells from maize anthers, which greatly promoted studies on plant anther scRNA-seq [40]. The comparative studies on transcriptomic dynamics between different types of cells facilitate the deeper understanding of functions of specific cell layers on anther development.

### 3.4 Different treatments

At the reproductive stage, plant is more sensitive to external environment conditions. The abiotic stresses, such as high temperature, drought, and cold and freezing stresses, will critically affect the developmental process of anther and pollen in flowing plants. Though there have been numerous studies on stress resistance and response in plant, the regulatory pathways of stress response and their cross talk at molecular level should be further investigated for anther development. Additionally, more effective stress-resistant genes should be identified for the purpose of crop improvement. Plant comparative transcriptomics between normal and stress-treated plants provide a wide insight into the stress response mechanisms of plant during sexual reproductive stage. Zhang et al. investigated the genome-wide transcriptional changes of rice panicle under heat treatment (40°C) and found thousands of DEGs participating in transcriptional regulation, transport, cellular homeostasis, and stress response [41]. Studies on photosensitive or thermosensitive GMS lines can also reveal a lot of genes responding to environmental changes.

## 4. A case study: revealing the molecular functions of a MS gene, *ZmMs33*, by comparative transcriptomics

The discoveries of genes that play key roles in the development of maize anther provide important genetic resources for the utilization of heterosis in maize. Analysis of functional mechanism of GMS genes can effectively promote researches on anther development biology and deepen our understanding of molecular mechanism controlling sexual plant reproduction [42]. There are several published case studies containing comparative transcriptomics analysis on maize GMS genes in our laboratory, including *ZmMs7* [43], *ZmMs20* [44], *ZmMs30* [45], and *ZmMs33* [46, 47]. We used comparative transcriptomics analysis based on developmental anthers of *ZmMs33* wild type and *ms33–6038* mutant to analyze the transcription changes corresponding to male sterility phenotype and to further investigate the underlying molecular mechanisms of GMS regulated by *ZmMs33* gene.

This *ms33–6038* mutant is complete male sterility and displays small and pale-yellow anthers (**Figure 3A**). Transmission electron microscope (TEM) observation and dynamic scanning electron microscopy (SEM) analysis were performed to analyze the phenotypic alteration of anther wall layers, microspores, Ubisch bodies, and exine between wild type and *ms33–6038* mutant during anther developmental stages (**Figure 3A–C**).

Maize *Zm00001d007714* was identified as *ZmMs33* via a map-based cloning approach (**Figure 3D**). *ZmMs33* encodes an esterase that belongs to gene family of glycerol-3-phosphate acyltransferase (GPAT) in maize. To further confirm gene function of *Zm00001d007714*, a CRISPR/Cas9 system was used to generate targeted knockout lines. Three types of $T_0$-generation maize plants homozygous for null alleles of *Zm00001d007714* were observed to be complete male sterility (**Figure 3E**), suggesting that function loss of *Zm00001d007714* is the causal mutation for male sterile phenotype of the *ms33* mutant.

Subsequently, RNA-seq was performed using anther tissues during developmental stages 5–9 to obtain a comprehensive transcriptional profile of WT and *ms33-6038*. Three biological samples were collected at each developmental stage for sequencing. After data preparation and transcription level estimation, we compared similarities of transcriptional profiles of protein-coding genes by principal component analysis (PCA) (**Figure 3F**) and found good repeatability among three biological repeats.

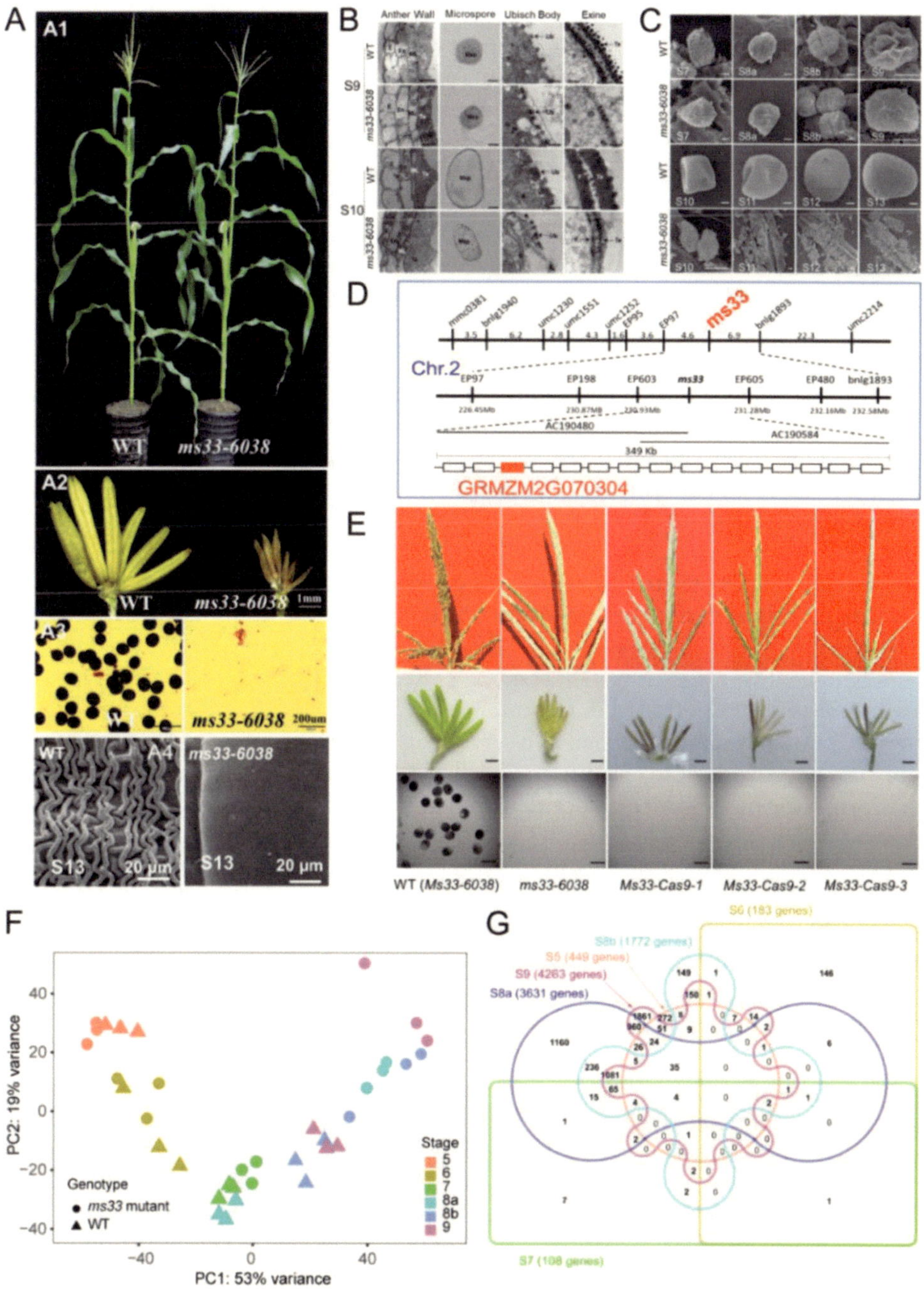


**Figure 3.**
*Reveal ZmMs33 gene functions for anther development by comparative transcriptomics analysis. (A) Phenotype of whole plants (A1), anthers (A2), pollen grains (A3), and outer surface of anther wall (A4) of WT and ms33–6038 mutant. (B) TEM analysis of anther wall layers, microspores, Ubisch bodies, and exine in WT and ms33–6038 mutant. (C) SEM analysis of microspores and pollen grains in WT and ms33–6038 mutant. (D) Map-based cloning of ZmMs33 gene. (E) Phenotypes of tassels, anthers, and pollen grains in three ms33 knockout lines generated by a CRISPR/Cas9 system. (F) PCA analysis of RNA-seq data from WT and ms33–6038 mutant. (G) Venn plot of DEGs at each developmental stage.* ***Figure 3A–C*** *was cited from [46].* ***Figure 3D*** *and* ***E*** *was cited from [47].*

Finally, we identified DEGs between WT and mutant and between adjacent developmental stages, separately. We found that the amount of DEGs between WT and mutant at stages 5–7 was significantly smaller in magnitude than that at stages 8a–9 (**Figure 3G**), indicating that *ms33* mutant transcriptomes are significantly divergent from WT starting from stage 8a. The transcriptome landscapes of WT were similar to those of *ms33* mutant at stages 5–7. Besides, DEG amounts were various between adjacent developmental stages. It is worth noting that the DEG amount between WT and mutant exceeded that between adjacent stages from stage 8a–9. This result implied that the transcriptomes were significantly changed at the later three stages. Therefore, we compared the transcriptomes between genotypes at the former three and the later three stages, separately. In contrast to a limited number of DEGs (only two genes) shared by the former three stages, there were thousands of shared DEGs at the later three stages. GSE analysis based on KEGG database suggested that the upregulated gene set was firstly enriched in the function of biosynthesis of secondary metabolites, while the downregulated genes were significantly related to the photosynthesis process. This pathway enrichment analysis partly represents the alterations in metabolisms and physiological activities closely associated with the transcriptional changes caused by function defect of *ms33*.

## 5. Gene co-expression and regulatory networks reconstructed by comparative transcriptomics method

Though DEGs are mainly identified by pairwise comparisons between transcriptomes of tissues, stages, or treatment conditions and can reflect most of the transcriptional changes between two sets of samples, these transcriptional alterations are not sufficient to explain the detailed molecular mechanism underlying tissue-specific development processes and stress-resistant pathways. Moreover, the molecular functions of genes act under GRNs. All the biological processes of growth, development, stress response, and reproduction are regulated by GRNs. The prediction of gene regulatory relationships and the reconstruction of the GRNs by using the transcriptome data are also the major aims in transcriptomics studies, except for the DGEP and DEG analyses.

### 5.1 Gene co-expression analysis

Function-related genes tend to co-express in a cell, either to form a complex or to involve in the same biological pathway. Thus, the similar pattern of gene expressions can be used as an indicator to predict gene functions. Gene co-expression (GCE) analysis is a powerful tool to discover important functional genes in biological processes including anther development. A relatively early study identified two functional GMS genes, *POLYKETIDE SYNTHASE A* (*PKSA*) and *PKSB*, through detecting co-expressed genes with *ACOS5*, a GMS gene belonging to fatty acyl-CoA synthetase gene family, based on microarray data in *A. thaliana* [48]. Similarly, *ABORTED MICROSPORES* (*AMS*) gene was reported participating in the pollen wall formation in rice by the analyses of 98 co-expressed genes with *AMS* in flower development [49]. GCE analysis can be also used to investigate the biological functions and the regulatory targets of a gene. This genome-wide analysis on GCE networks has been performed based on microarray data from *A. thaliana* anther tissues, and 254 complete GCE groups containing 10,513 anther-transcribed genes were revealed [50]. Another microarray-based GCE network was reconstructed in *A. thaliana* anther by using 10,797 genes expressed in anther/flora, and transcriptional landscape of GMS mutant was included in the stable examination of this newly constructed network [51]. In rice, microarrays from WT anther tissue across stages 2–14 and nine GMS lines were integrated to reconstruct a big GCE network containing more than 9000 genes and 0.4 million pairs of co-expression relationships [52].

RNA-seq data-based GCE network analysis was performed in anther when high-throughput sequencing technology was developed. In woodland strawberry, stages 1–12 floral samples dissected by LCM or hand, including stages 6–12 anther tissues, were sequenced by RNA-seq. Gene co-expression network analysis was used to reconstruct GCE networks in strawberry's flower development, and 23 modules were discovered from the GCE networks including 4584 pollen-specific genes [34]. These genome-wide GCE networks are useful for characterization of genes associated with anther development and floral reproduction.

### 5.2 TF-encoding gene regulatory network

Genes with their products forming one protein complex, genes encoding transcription factor (TF) and TF target genes, and genes functioning in the same metabolic pathway or stress-resistant process often tend to be co-expressed in a cell. Therefore, the expression-associated genes in GCE network may be not directly functionally linked. A more accurate and robust gene regulatory network is needed for both the biological function and network researches at molecular and genome levels. One way to improve the gene regulatory network is to introduce gene regulatory types into the network. Several TF gene regulatory networks (TF-GRN), also called as transcriptional regulatory network (TRN), were reconstructed based on expression patterns of TF-encoding genes and TF target genes from transcriptome data. One TF-GRN comprised 19 TFs and their 101 target genes involving in *A. thaliana* pollen development [53]. Another GRN of early anther development was constructed by interactively analyzing transcriptome data from three GMS lines of TF-encoding gene knockout mutants [9]. In the maize genome, there are 2298 TF-encoding genes identified which belonged to 56 diverse families [54]. A total of 3078 TF-encoding genes belonging to 59 families are predicted in silico analysis in rice genome [55]. These TF databases, combining with increased amount of transcriptome data from mutants of TF-encoding genes and other omics data (e.g., Chip-seq, DAP-seq), provide abundant data for the reconstruction of TF-GRN with increased credibility, applicability, and completeness.

### 5.3 miRNA target gene regulatory network

Both transcriptional and posttranscriptional regulations are crucial in controlling the normal development and stress-resistant process in cellular life. The miRNA-mediated regulation model on target genes is a well-studied posttranscriptional gene regulation pathway that plays important roles in floral identification and the following development of flower organs [56–58] as well as male fertility [59, 60]. Beyond numerous case studies on functional miRNAs in anther development and GMS genes [61–64], the expression profile of miRNAs and the regulatory networks were investigated to elevate our understanding on the transcriptional regulatory mechanism of miRNAs. GRNs between miRNA and their target genes have been constructed via flower/anther transcriptomics in the model plant species, *A. thaliana*, and some other plants [65–68]. Furthermore, comparative transcriptomics analysis on small miRNAs has been commonly used as a research method to reveal the transcriptional alterations between fertility and sterility lines in economic and food plant species, such as maize [45], tomato [69], cotton [70, 71], wheat [72, 73], pine [74], lycium [75], watermelon [32], and *Brassica campestris* [76].

### 5.4 ceRNA-miRNA regulatory network

It is well known that miRNAs are crucial regulators on gene expressions that control key biological functions including anther development, since miRNA was firstly found in nematodes in 1993 [77]. It is noteworthy that a novel type of gene regulatory model, the competing endogenous RNA (ceRNA) hypothesis, was recently proposed [78]. According to the ceRNA hypothesis, some endogenous transcripts have abilities to adsorb miRNA molecules; subsequently, the expression levels of miRNA target genes can be derepressed [78, 79]. A typical ceRNA in plant, a long noncoding RNA, *IPSI*, was found in *A. thaliana*. It could completely sponge miRNA *ath-miR399* and indirectly increase the transcription levels of an important gene involved in phosphate homeostasis [80]. The following studies revealed that transcripts of protein-coding genes, pseudogene, transposable elements, simple sequence repeat, and circular RNAs have molecular functions as ceRNAs [79, 81, 82], indicating that the ceRNA-miRNA relationship is an essential gene regulatory mechanism in the growth and development of plants and animals. Consequently, it is necessary to introduce ceRNA regulators into GRN construction. Here, we present our recent study on reconstructing ceRNA regulatory network mainly based on RNA-seq and small RNA-seq transcriptomes from developmental maize anther.

## 6. A case study: reconstructing ceRNA-miRNA target gene regulatory networks using transcriptome data of maize anther

Here we summarized the research progress of one recently completed research related to the ceRNA-mediated GRN in our laboratory. Generally speaking, this is the first study introducing ceRNA regulation into miRNA target gene regulatory pathway for deeply dissecting the mechanism of anther development and sexual plant reproduction at a network level. This provides a fresh example for GRN research by plant comparative transcriptomics and has dual significance in both theoretical and practical senses. It may also provide new thoughts and strategies for further transcriptome-based GRN studies.

It is well known that gene expressions are controlled by the GRN in cellular life. Newly found regulatory patterns (e.g., miRNA pathway and epigenetic modification) have enhanced our understanding on the GRN. Recently, "ceRNA hypothesis" was proposed as a novel type of gene regulatory relationship and was found to participate in different development and stress response processes of organisms by a number of case studies. However, the network level study on ceRNA regulatory functions is still rare, which limited our deep understanding on the GRN. In addition, studies on the GRN of sexual plant reproduction and male sterility are crucial for both fundamental biological significance and applications in plant hybrid breeding and seed production. We investigated ceRNA-miRNA target gene regulatory network in maize anther developmental process by plant comparative transcriptomics method. Six steps were performed from raw sequencing data preparation to the finally constructed GRN (**Figure 4**). *Firstly*, we performed RNA- and small RNA-seq using anther tissues at three developmental stages from two maize lines to obtain a relative broad transcriptional landscape in anther development and transcribed loci that are stably expressed in maize species. *Secondly*, we identified stably transcribed loci based on the maize reference genome and estimated their transcription levels. In this step, we only used shared transcription loci identified from RNA-seq data between two maize lines (**Figure 4A**). Notably, these transcribed loci were divided into five groups such as protein-coding genes, lncRNAs, transposable elements, and unassigned loci. *Thirdly*, we identified known miRNAs

*DOI: http://dx.doi.org/10.5772/intechopen.88318*

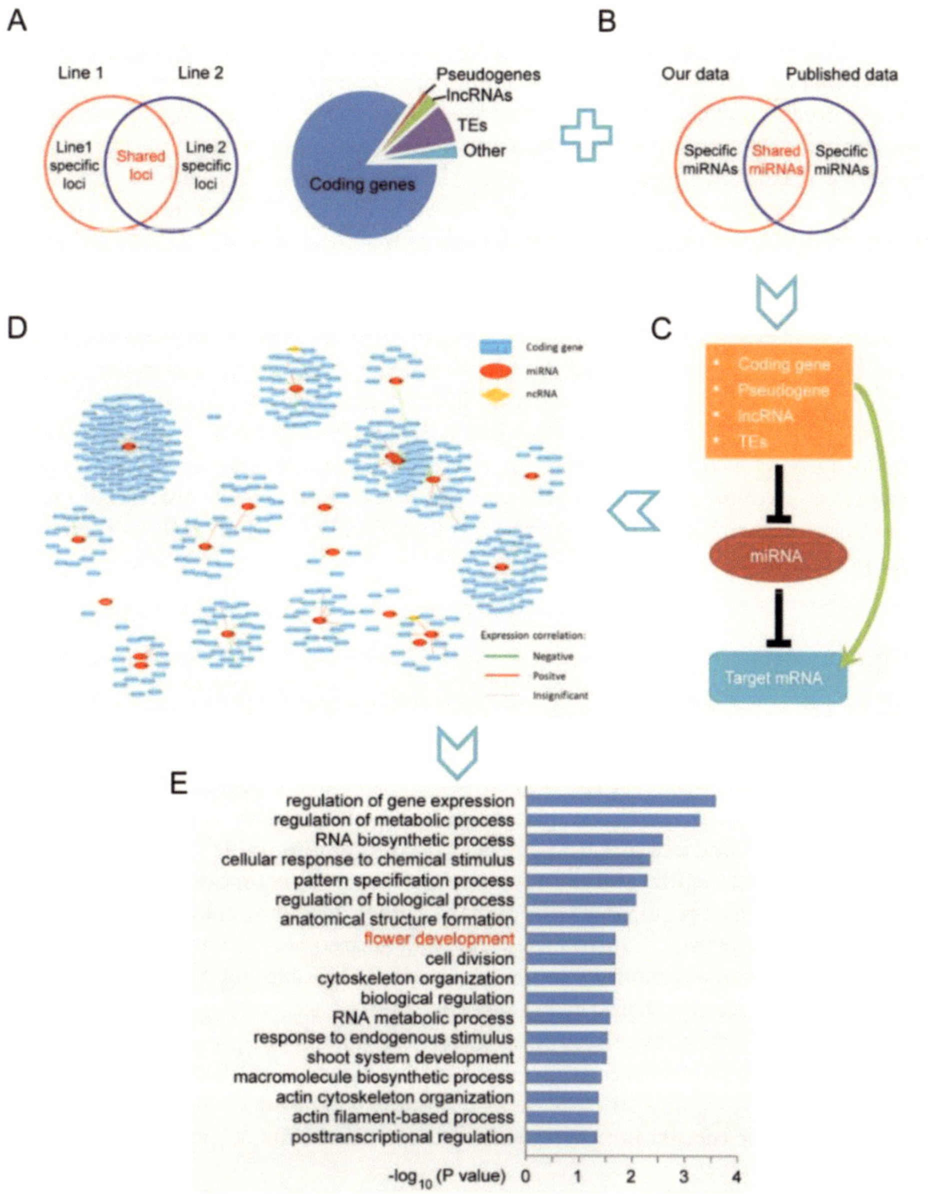


**Figure 4.**
*A flowchart of reconstructing the ceRNA-miRNA target gene regulatory network in developmental maize anther. (A) Identification and classification of stably transcribed loci in maize anther. (B) Identification of known miRNA in maize anther. (C) Prediction of ceRNA-miRNA and miRNA target gene interaction pairs. (D) Reconstruction of ceRNA-miRNA target gene regulatory networks. (E) GSE analysis of target genes in the networks.*

and predicted potential novel miRNAs that may be involved in maize anther development. Sequenced small RNA data were obtained from the same samples that were used in RNA-seq. A matched dataset (e.g., matched RNA and small RNA sequenced dataset here) is important in experimental design and more powerful to reveal the investigated biological questions. Though the analysis workflow of small RNA-seq data is similar to that of RNA-seq data in general (**Figure 1**), there are some differences between them. In our analysis, we reanalyzed two sets of published small RNA data to compare with their results from our own sequenced data for credible known and potential novel miRNAs involved in maize anther development [23, 83] (**Figure 4B**). This is an important check method to confirm the stability of research results and conclusions. *Fourthly*, we predicted ceRNA-miRNA interaction pairs and miRNA target gene regulatory pairs by computational approach (**Figure 4C**). Bioinformatics analysis in this step is mainly based on genome sequence but not the transcriptomes. *Fifthly*, we reconstructed ceRNA-miRNA target gene regulatory networks by predicted interaction pairs and transcription correlation patterns from transcriptomics data (**Figure 4D**). It is well known that miRNAs could repress the transcription levels of their target genes. Additionally, ceRNA was demonstrated to negatively regulate the transcription levels of matched miRNAs. The negatively associated gene pairs in transcription levels may be more credible in mutual interactions. By integrating ceRNA-miRNA and miRNA target gene interactions, we reconstructed ceRNA-miRNA target gene regulatory networks in maize anther. *Finally*, we generally investigated the functional significance of genes in the regulatory network by GO enrichment analysis. In these networks, we found a number of well-studied genes and miRNA target gene pairs involved in maize anther development and male sterility, suggesting that the ceRNA-miRNA target gene regulatory networks contribute to anther development in maize. Besides, GO analysis of target genes in the network revealed that they are functionally enriched in flower development process (**Figure 4E**) [84].

## 7. Conclusions

Here, we summarized major points in comparative transcriptomics analysis from the commonly utilized workflow to the closely related research cases and from the single gene-based function analysis to GRN-based gene function investigation. In GMS gene studies, the research experiments using comparative transcriptomics method to investigate key functional genes and the genome-wide GRNs in developmental anther will facilitate our systematical understanding on the biological processes and molecular regulatory networks for anther development and sexual plant reproduction. More importantly, case studies illustrated here have a general meaning on technologies and methodologies for functional researches of other biological pathways and processes. With the fast advancement of sequencing technology, plant comparative transcriptomics has achieved considerable development. However, our understanding on the transcriptional dynamics and gene regulatory relationships of biological processes are far from being completed. Consequently, more efforts are needed for the further improvement of comparative transcriptomics in plant biological studies.

## Acknowledgements

The research in our lab was supported by the National Key Research and Development Program of China (2018YFD0100806, 2017YFD0102001, 2017YFD0101201), the National Transgenic Major Program of China (2018ZX0800922B, 2018ZX0801006B), the National Natural Science Foundation of China (31,771,875, 31,871,702), the Fundamental Research Funds for the Central Universities of China (06500060), and the "Ten Thousand Plan" of National High-level Talents Special Support Plan (For Xiangyuan Wan).

## Conflict of interest

The authors declare that they have no conflict of interest.

## Abbreviations

| | |
|---|---|
| ceRNA | competing endogenous RNA |
| DE | differentially expressed |
| DGEP | digital gene expression profile |
| GCE | gene co-expression |
| GEG | differentially expressed gene |
| GEM | gene expression microarray |
| GMS | genic male sterility |
| GO | gene ontology |
| GRN | gene regulatory network |
| GSE | gene set enrichment |
| KEGG | Kyoto encyclopedia of genes and genomes |
| LCM | laser capture microdissection |
| LncRNA | long noncoding RNA |
| miRNA | microRNA |
| MPSS | massively parallel signature sequencing |
| MS | male sterility |
| NGS | the next-generation sequencing |
| RNA-seq | RNA sequencing |
| SAGE | serial analysis of gene expression |
| scRNA-seq | single-cell RNA sequencing |
| SEM | scanning electron microscopy |
| TEM | transmission electron microscope |
| TF | transcription factor |
| TF-GRN | TF gene regulatory network |
| TRN | transcriptional regulatory network |
| WT | wild type |

## Author details

Xiangyuan Wan[1,2]* and Ziwen Li[1,2]*

1 Biology and Agriculture Research Center, University of Science and Technology Beijing, Beijing, China

2 Beijing Engineering Laboratory of Main Crop Bio-Tech Breeding, Beijing International Science and Technology Cooperation Base of Bio-Tech Breeding, Beijing Solidwill Sci-Tech Co. Ltd., Beijing, China

*Address all correspondence to: wanxiangyuan@ustb.edu.cn and liziwen@ustb.edu.cn

## References

[1] Crick F. Central dogma of molecular biology. Nature. 1970;**227**:561-563

[2] Schena M, Shalon D, Davis RW, Brown PO. Quantitative monitoring of gene expression patterns with a complementary DNA microarray. Science. 1995;**270**:467-470

[3] Byron SA, Van Keuren-Jensen KR, Engelthaler DM, Carpten JD, Craig DW. Translating RNA sequencing into clinical diagnostics: Opportunities and challenges. Nature Reviews. Genetics. 2016;**17**:257-271

[4] Velculescu VE, Zhang L, Vogelstein B, Kinzler KW. Serial analysis of gene expression. Science. 1995;**270**:484-487

[5] Brenner S, Johnson M, Bridgham J, Golda G, Lloyd DH, Johnson D, et al. Gene expression analysis by massively parallel signature sequencing (MPSS) on microbead arrays. Nature Biotechnology. 2000;**18**:630-634

[6] Stelpflug SC, Sekhon RS, Vaillancourt B, Hirsch CN, Buell CR, de Leon N, et al. An expanded maize gene expression atlas based on RNA sequencing and its use to explore root development. Plant Genome. 2016;**9**:1-15

[7] Xing S, Zachgo S. ROXY1 and ROXY2, two Arabidopsis glutaredoxin genes, are required for anther development. The Plant Journal. 2008;**53**:790-801

[8] Feng B, Lu D, Ma X, Peng Y, Sun Y, Ning G, et al. Regulation of the Arabidopsis anther transcriptome by DYT1 for pollen development. The Plant Journal. 2012;**72**:612-624

[9] Ma X, Feng B, Ma H. AMS-dependent and independent regulation of anther transcriptome and comparison with those affected by other Arabidopsis anther genes. BMC Plant Biology. 2012;**12**:23

[10] Xu J, Yang C, Yuan Z, Zhang D, Gondwe MY, Ding Z, et al. The aborted microspores regulatory network is required for postmeiotic male reproductive development in *Arabidopsis thaliana*. Plant Cell. 2010;**22**:91-107

[11] Wijeratne AJ, Zhang W, Sun Y, Liu W, Albert R, Zheng Z, et al. Differential gene expression in Arabidopsis wild-type and mutant anthers: Insights into anther cell differentiation and regulatory networks. The Plant Journal. 2007;**52**:14-29

[12] Yang C, Vizcay-Barrena G, Conner K, Wilson ZA. Male sterility1 is required for tapetal development and pollen wall biosynthesis. Plant Cell. 2007;**19**:3530-3548

[13] Alves-Ferreira M, Wellmer F, Banhara A, Kumar V, Riechmann JL, et al. Global expression profiling applied to the analysis of Arabidopsis stamen development. Plant Physiology. 2007;**145**:747-762

[14] Wei D, Liu M, Chen H, Zheng Y, Liu Y, Wang X, et al. Inducer of CBF expression 1 is a male fertility regulator impacting anther dehydration in Arabidopsis. PLoS Genetics. 2018;**14**:e1007695

[15] Lu P, Chai M, Yang J, Ning G, Wang G, Ma H. The Arabidopsis callose defective microspore1 gene is required for male fertility through regulating callose metabolism during microsporogenesis. Plant Physiology. 2014;**164**:1893-1904

[16] Lou Y, Xu XF, Zhu J, Gu JN, Blackmore S, Yang ZN. The tapetal AHL family protein TEK determines nexine formation in the pollen wall. Nature Communications. 2014;**5**:3855

[17] Zhu E, You C, Wang S, Cui J, Niu B, Wang Y, et al. The DYT1-interacting proteins bHLH010, bHLH089 and bHLH091 are redundantly required for Arabidopsis anther development and transcriptome. The Plant Journal. 2015;**83**:976-990

[18] Li H, Yuan Z, Vizcay-Barrena G, Yang C, Liang W, Zong J, et al. Persistent tapetal cell1 encodes a PHD-finger protein that is required for tapetal cell death and pollen development in rice. Plant Physiology. 2011;**156**:615-630

[19] Jung KH, Han MJ, Lee YS, Kim YW, Hwang I, Kim MJ, et al. Rice undeveloped tapetum1 is a major regulator of early tapetum development. Plant Cell. 2005;**17**:2705-2722

[20] Aya K, Ueguchi-Tanaka M, Kondo M, Hamada K, Yano K, Nishimura M, et al. Gibberellin modulates anther development in rice via the transcriptional regulation of GAMYB. Plant Cell. 2009;**21**:1453-1472

[21] Zhang DS, Liang WQ, Yuan Z, Li N, Shi J, Wang J, et al. Tapetum degeneration retardation is critical for aliphatic metabolism and gene regulation during rice pollen development. Molecular Plant. 2008;**1**:599-610

[22] Hu L, Liang W, Yin C, Cui X, Zong J, Wang X, et al. Rice MADS3 regulates ROS homeostasis during late anther development. Plant Cell. 2011;**23**:515-533

[23] Nan GL, Zhai J, Arikit S, Morrow D, Fernandes J, Mai L, et al. MS23, a master basic helix-loop-helix factor, regulates the specification and development of the tapetum in maize. Development. 2017;**144**:163-172

[24] Zhang H, Egger RL, Kelliher T, Morrow D, Fernandes J, Nan GL, et al. Transcriptomes and proteomes define gene expression progression in pre-meiotic maize anthers. G3 (Bethesda). 2014;**4**:993-1010

[25] Wang Z, Li J, Chen S, Heng Y, Chen Z, Yang J, et al. Poaceae-specific MS1 encodes a phospholipid-binding protein for male fertility in bread wheat. Proceedings of the National Academy of Sciences of the United States of America. 2017;**114**:12614-12,619

[26] Ni F, Qi J, Hao Q, Lyu B, Luo MC, Wang Y, et al. Wheat Ms2 encodes for an orphan protein that confers male sterility in grass species. Nature Communications. 2017;**8**:15121

[27] Jeong HJ, Kang JH, Zhao M, Kwon JK, Choi HS, Bae JH, et al. Tomato male sterile 1035 is essential for pollen development and meiosis in anthers. Journal of Experimental Botany. 2014;**65**:6693-6709

[28] Omidvar V, Mohorianu I, Dalmay T, Zheng Y, Fei Z, Pucci A, et al. Transcriptional regulation of male-sterility in 7B-1 male-sterile tomato mutant. PLoS One. 2017;**12**:e0170715

[29] Qu C, Fu F, Liu M, Zhao H, Liu C, Li J, et al. Comparative transcriptome analysis of recessive male sterility (RGMS) in sterile and fertile *Brassica napus* lines. PLoS One. 2015;**10**:e0144118

[30] Liu XQ, Liu ZQ, Yu CY, Dong JG, Hu SW, Xu AX. TGMS in rapeseed (*Brassica napus*) resulted in aberrant transcriptional regulation, asynchronous microsporocyte meiosis, defective tapetum, and fused sexine. Frontiers in Plant Science. 2017;**8**:1268

[31] Yan X, Zeng X, Wang S, Li K, Yuan R, Gao H, et al. Aberrant meiotic prophase I leads to genic male sterility in the novel TE5A mutant of *Brassica napus*. Scientific Reports. 2016;**6**:33955

[32] Rhee SJ, Seo M, Jang YJ, Cho S, Lee GP. Transcriptome profiling of differentially expressed genes in floral

buds and flowers of male sterile and fertile lines in watermelon. BMC Genomics. 2015;**16**:914

[33] Ma J, Skibbe DS, Fernandes J, Walbot V. Male reproductive development: Gene expression profiling of maize anther and pollen ontogeny. Genome Biology. 2008;**9**:R181

[34] Hollender CA, Kang C, Darwish O, Geretz A, Matthews BF, Slovin J, et al. Floral transcriptomes in woodland strawberry uncover developing receptacle and anther gene networks. Plant Physiology. 2014;**165**:1062-1075

[35] Yue L, Twell D, Kuang Y, Liao J, Zhou X. Transcriptome analysis of *Hamelia patens* (Rubiaceae) anthers reveals candidate genes for tapetum and pollen wall development. Frontiers in Plant Science. 2016;**7**:1991

[36] Chen Z, Rao P, Yang X, Su X, Zhao T, Gao K, et al. A global view of transcriptome dynamics during male floral bud development in *Populus tomentosa*. Scientific Reports. 2018;**8**:722

[37] Ma Y, Kang J, Wu J, Zhu Y, Wang X. Identification of tapetum-specific genes by comparing global gene expression of four different male sterile lines in *Brassica oleracea*. Plant Molecular Biology. 2015;**87**:541-554

[38] Hirano K, Aya K, Hobo T, Sakakibara H, Kojima M, Shim RA, et al. Comprehensive transcriptome analysis of phytohormone biosynthesis and signaling genes in microspore/pollen and tapetum of rice. Plant and Cell Physiology. 2008;**49**:1429-1450

[39] Yuan TL, Huang WJ, He J, Zhang D, Tang WH. Stage-specific gene profiling of germinal cells helps delineate the mitosis/meiosis transition. Plant Physiology. 2018;**176**:1610-1626

[40] Nelms B, Walbot V. Defining the developmental program leading to meiosis in maize. Science. 2019;**364**:52-56

[41] Zhang X, Li J, Liu A, Zou J, Zhou X, Xiang J, et al. Expression profile in rice panicle: Insights into heat response mechanism at reproductive stage. PLoS One. 2012;**7**:e49652

[42] Wan X, Wu S, Li Z, Dong Z, An X, Ma B, et al. Maize genic male-sterility genes and their applications in hybrid breeding: Progress and perspectives. Molecular Plant. 2019;**12**:321-342

[43] Zhang D, Wu S, An X, Xie K, Dong Z, Zhou Y, et al. Construction of a multicontrol sterility system for a maize male-sterile line and hybrid seed production based on the ZmMs7 gene encoding a PHD-finger transcription factor. Plant Biotechnology Journal. 2018;**16**:459-471

[44] Wang Y, Liu D, Tian Y, Wu S, An X, Dong Z, et al. Map-based cloning, phylogenetic, and microsynteny analyses of ZmMs20 gene regulating male fertility in maize. International Journal of Molecular Sciences. 2019;**20**:1411

[45] An X, Dong Z, Tian Y, Xie K, Wu S, Zhu T, et al. ZmMs30 encoding a novel GDSL lipase is essential for male fertility and valuable for hybrid breeding in maize. Molecular Plant. 2019;**12**:343-359

[46] Zhu T, Wu S, Zhang D, Li Z, Xie K, An X, et al. Genome-wide analysis of maize GPAT gene family and cytological characterization and breeding application of ZmMs33/ZmGPAT6 gene. Theoretical and Applied Genetics. 2019;**132**:2137-2154

[47] Xie K, Wu S, Li Z, Zhou Y, Zhang D, Dong Z, et al. Map-based cloning and characterization of Zea mays male sterility33 (ZmMs33) gene, encoding a

glycerol-3-phosphate acyltransferase. Theoretical and Applied Genetics. 2018;**131**:1363-1378

[48] Kim SS, Grienenberger E, Lallemand B, Colpitts CC, Kim SY, Souza Cde A, et al. LAP6/polyketide synthase A and LAP5/polyketide synthase B encode hydroxyalkyl alpha-pyrone synthases required for pollen development and sporopollenin biosynthesis in *Arabidopsis thaliana*. Plant Cell. 2010;**22**:4045-4066

[49] Xu J, Ding Z, Vizcay-Barrena G, Shi J, Liang W, Yuan Z, et al. Aborted microspores acts as a master regulator of pollen wall formation in Arabidopsis. Plant Cell. 2014;**26**:1544-1556

[50] Jiao QJ, Huang Y, Shen HB. Large-scale mining co-expressed genes in Arabidopsis anther: From pair to group. Computational Biology and Chemistry. 2011;**35**:62-68

[51] Pearce S, Ferguson A, King J, Wilson ZA. FlowerNet: A gene expression correlation network for anther and pollen development. Plant Physiology. 2015;**167**:1717-1730

[52] Lin H, Yu J, Pearce SP, Zhang D, Wilson ZA. RiceAntherNet: A gene co-expression network for identifying anther and pollen development genes. The Plant Journal. 2017;**92**:1076-1091

[53] Wang J, Qiu X, Li Y, Deng Y, Shi T. A transcriptional dynamic network during *Arabidopsis thaliana* pollen development. BMC Systems Biology. 2011;**5**(Suppl 3):S8

[54] Jiang Y, Zeng B, Zhao H, Zhang M, Xie S, Lai J. Genome-wide transcription factor gene prediction and their expressional tissue-specificities in maize. Journal of Integrative Plant Biology. 2012;**54**:616-630

[55] Chen W, Chen Z, Luo F, Liao M, Wei S, Yang Z, et al. RicetissueTFDB: A genome-wide identification of tissue-specific transcription factors in rice. Plant Genome. 2019;**12**:1-11

[56] Luo Y, Guo Z, Li L. Evolutionary conservation of microRNA regulatory programs in plant flower development. Developmental Biology. 2013;**380**:133-144

[57] Li X. Next-generation sequencing sheds new light on small RNAs in plant reproductive development. Current Issues in Molecular Biology. 2018;**27**:143-170

[58] Li ZF, Zhang YC, Chen YQ. miRNAs and lncRNAs in reproductive development. Plant Science. 2015;**238**:46-52

[59] Ru P, Xu L, Ma H, Huang H. Plant fertility defects induced by the enhanced expression of microRNA167. Cell Research. 2006;**16**:457-465

[60] Chuck G, Meeley R, Irish E, Sakai H, Hake S. The maize tasselseed4 microRNA controls sex determination and meristem cell fate by targeting Tasselseed6/indeterminate spikelet1. Nature Genetics. 2007;**39**:1517-1521

[61] Millar AA, Gubler F. The Arabidopsis GAMYB-like genes, MYB33 and MYB65, are microRNA-regulated genes that redundantly facilitate anther development. Plant Cell. 2005;**17**:705-721

[62] Ding Y, Ma Y, Liu N, Xu J, Hu Q, Li Y, et al. MicroRNAs involved in auxin signaling modulate male sterility under high-temperature stress in cotton (*Gossypium hirsutum*). The Plant Journal. 2017;**91**:977-994

[63] Field S, Thompson B. Analysis of the maize dicer-like1 mutant, fuzzy tassel, implicates microRNAs in anther maturation and dehiscence. PLoS One. 2016;**11**:e0146534

[64] Xing S, Salinas M, Hohmann S, Berndtgen R, Huijser P. miR156-targeted and nontargeted SBP-box transcription factors act in concert to secure male fertility in Arabidopsis. Plant Cell. 2010;**22**:3935-3950

[65] Feng N, Song G, Guan J, Chen K, Jia M, Huang D, et al. Transcriptome profiling of wheat inflorescence development from spikelet initiation to floral patterning identified stage-specific regulatory genes. Plant Physiology. 2017;**174**:1779-1794

[66] Chen J, Su P, Chen P, Li Q, Yuan X, Liu Z. Insights into the cotton anther development through association analysis of transcriptomic and small RNA sequencing. BMC Plant Biology. 2018;**18**:154

[67] Srivastava S, Zheng Y, Kudapa H, Jagadeeswaran G, Hivrale V, Varshney RK, et al. High throughput sequencing of small RNA component of leaves and inflorescence revealed conserved and novel miRNAs as well as phasiRNA loci in chickpea. Plant Science. 2015;**235**:46-57

[68] Wei LQ, Yan LF, Wang T. Deep sequencing on genome-wide scale reveals the unique composition and expression patterns of microRNAs in developing pollen of *Oryza sativa*. Genome Biology. 2011;**12**:R53

[69] Omidvar V, Mohorianu I, Dalmay T, Fellner M. Identification of miRNAs with potential roles in regulation of anther development and male-sterility in 7B-1 male-sterile tomato mutant. BMC Genomics. 2015;**16**:878

[70] Yang X, Zhao Y, Xie D, Sun Y, Zhu X, Esmaeili N, et al. Identification and functional analysis of microRNAs involved in the anther development in cotton genic male sterile line Yu98-8A. International Journal of Molecular Sciences. 2016;**17**:1677

[71] Wei M, Wei H, Wu M, Song M, Zhang J, Yu J, et al. Comparative expression profiling of miRNA during anther development in genetic male sterile and wild type cotton. BMC Plant Biology. 2013;**13**:66

[72] Sun L, Sun G, Shi C, Sun D. Transcriptome analysis reveals new microRNAs-mediated pathway involved in anther development in male sterile wheat. BMC Genomics. 2018;**19**:333

[73] Tang Z, Zhang L, Xu C, Yuan S, Zhang F, Zheng Y, et al. Uncovering small RNA-mediated responses to cold stress in a wheat thermosensitive genic male-sterile line by deep sequencing. Plant Physiology. 2012;**159**:721-738

[74] Niu SH, Liu C, Yuan HW, Li P, Li Y, Li W. Identification and expression profiles of sRNAs and their biogenesis and action-related genes in male and female cones of *Pinus tabuliformis*. BMC Genomics. 2015;**16**:693

[75] Shi J, Chen L, Zheng R, Guan C, Wang Y, Liang W, et al. Comparative phenotype and microRNAome in developing anthers of wild-type and male-sterile *Lycium barbarum* L. Plant Science. 2018;**274**:349-359

[76] Jiang J, Lv M, Liang Y, Ma Z, Cao J. Identification of novel and conserved miRNAs involved in pollen development in *Brassica campestris* ssp. chinensis by high-throughput sequencing and degradome analysis. BMC Genomics. 2014;**15**:146

[77] Lee RC, Feinbaum RL, Ambros V. The *C. elegans* heterochronic gene lin-4 encodes small RNAs with antisense complementarity to lin-14. Cell. 1993;**75**:843-854

[78] Salmena L, Poliseno L, Tay Y, Kats L, Pandolfi PP. A ceRNA hypothesis: The rosetta stone of a hidden RNA language? Cell. 2011;**146**:353-358

[79] Thomson DW, Dinger ME. Endogenous microRNA sponges: Evidence and controversy. Nature Reviews. Genetics. 2016;**17**:272-283

[80] Franco-Zorrilla JM, Valli A, Todesco M, Mateos I, Puga MI, Rubio-Somoza I, et al. Target mimicry provides a new mechanism for regulation of microRNA activity. Nature Genetics. 2007;**39**:1033-1037

[81] Tay Y, Rinn J, Pandolfi PP. The multilayered complexity of ceRNA crosstalk and competition. Nature. 2014;**505**:344-352

[82] Paschoal AR, Lozada-Chavez I, Domingues DS, Stadler PF. ceRNAs in plants: Computational approaches and associated challenges for target mimic research. Briefings in Bioinformatics. 2018;**19**:1273-1289

[83] Zhai J, Zhang H, Arikit S, Huang K, Nan GL, Walbot V, et al. Spatiotemporally dynamic, cell-type-dependent premeiotic and meiotic phasiRNAs in maize anthers. Proceedings of the National Academy of Sciences of the United States of America. 2015;**112**:3146-3151

[84] Li Z, An X, Zhu T, Yan T, Wu S, Tian Y, et al. Discovering and constructing ceRNA-miRNA-target gene regulatory networks during anther development in maize. International Journal of Molecular Sciences. 2019;**20**:3480

Chapter 5

# Transcriptome Analysis for Abiotic Stresses in Rice (*Oryza sativa* L.)

*Ashutosh Kumar and Prasanta K. Dash*

## Abstract

Rice, a model monocot system, belongs to the family Poaceae and genus *Oryza*. Rice is the second largest produced cereal and staple food crop fulfilling the demand of half the world's population. Though rice demand is growing exponentially, its production is severely affected by variable environmental changes. The various abiotic factors drastically reduce the rice plant growth and yield by affecting its different growth stages. To fulfill the growing demand of rice, it is imperative to understand its molecular responses during stresses and to develop new varieties to overcome the stresses. Earlier, the microarray experiments have been used for the identification of coexpressive gene networks during various conditions in crop plants. Though the microarray experiments provided very useful information, the unviability of genome-wide information did not provide complete information about the regulatory gene networks involved in the stress response. The advancement of molecular techniques provided breakthrough to understanding the complex regulatory gene networks and their signaling pathways during stresses. The high-throughput RNA sequencing data have opened the floodgate of transcriptome data in rice. Here we have summarized some of the transcriptome data for abiotic molecular responses in rice, which further help to understand their complex regulatory mechanism.

**Keywords:** abiotic stresses, cold stress, drought, micronutrients, rice, RNA-Seq, salt stress, submergence, trace element stress, transcriptome

## 1. Introduction

Rice is the most important staple food crop across the globe and is a model monocot system [1]. It is the second largest produced cereal fulfilling the demand of half world's population. Rice belongs to family Poaceae and genus *Oryza*. Two species *Oryza sativa* (Asian rice) and *Oryza glaberrima* (African rice) out of 23 species have been cultivated worldwide [2]. The *O. sativa* is native to tropical and subtropical southern and southeastern Asia, while *O. glaberrima* is grown only in South Africa. A third species, *O. rufipogon*, has also been grown in South Asian, Chinese, New Guinean, Australian, and American farms. In Asia, *O. sativa* is separated into three subspecies according to its geographical environment: indica, japonica, and javanica. The variety indica refers to the tropical and subtropical varieties grown throughout South and Southeast Asia and Southern China. The variety japonica is grown in temperate areas of Japan, China, and Korea, while javanica varieties are grown alongside of indica in Indonesia (http://agropedia.iitk.ac.in/?q=content/botanical-classification-rice).

Rice is an annual plant, even though in tropical areas, it is cultivated perennially. It is self-pollinated (wind pollination) tropical C3 grass that evolved in a semi-aquatic, low-radiation habitat having arenchymatic tissues [3]. Rice is cultivated in more than 100 countries, with a total harvested area till 2017 is of approximately 165 million hectares, and produced ~700 million tons (503.9 million tons of milled rice) (http://www.fao.org/3/I9243EN/i9243en.pdf). About 91% of the rice in the world is grown in Asia (nearly 640 million tons) where 60% of the world's population lives. Rice is also cultivated in Sub-Saharan Africa and Latin Americas, and evenly poised in the Eastern and Western Asia. China and India, which account for more than one-third of global population, supply over half of the world's rice. The China produces ~30% of total world rice production followed by India (21%), Indonesia (9%), and Bangladesh (6%). On the other hand, rest of Asia, Americas, and Africa produce 37, 5, and 3%, respectively, of the total world rice production [4]. However, demand of the rice is still growing day by day, as the world population is mounting exponentially. To fulfill the demand of growing population, yield needs to be increased by the application of agricultural as well as biotechnological approaches.

Rice production is severely affected by changing environment including extreme variability in temperature and rainfall pattern along with other factors [5]. The abiotic stresses including drought, high salinity, high or low temperatures, flooding, high light, ozone, low nutrient availability, mineral deficiency, heavy metals, pollutants, wind and mechanical injury, drastically reduce the rice plant growth and yield by affecting it during different growth stages [6]. However, rice has very antagonistic character about tolerances and susceptibilities to abiotic stresses, as compared to other crops. It is very well known that rice paddy grows in standing water containing soil and can tolerate submergence at levels that would kill other crops. However, it is moderately tolerant to salinity and soil acidity but highly susceptible to drought and cold. Drought influences all physiological processes involved in plant growth and development [5]. Drought at vegetative stage can moderately reduce yield, but entire yield is lost if it occurs during pollen meiosis or fertilization [7]. The high salt concentration disrupts the ability of roots for efficient water uptake, leading to perturbation of crucial metabolic reactions inside the cell restricting plant growth and yield potential [8]. Low temperature reduces germination, causes poor establishment, delays phenological development, and increases spikelet sterility [9], and other physiological and metabolite changes causing low yield [10]. Furthermore, rice can tolerate partial submergence as paddy rice or deepwater rice because it is very well adapted to water-logged conditions as it has well-developed aerenchyma that facilitates oxygen diffusion and prevents anoxia in roots [11–13]. However, it was damaged when submerged partially or completely for a relatively longer period [14] due to the shortage of oxygen during submergence. The response of plants to low oxygen stress comprises complex biochemical and genetic programs that include the differential expressions of a large number of genes. Importantly, abiotic stress conditions not only harm the crop but also influence the manifestation and extent the pathogen infection, attack of insects, and growth of weeds [6]. Though rice has superior response to abiotic stresses, development of their improved tolerant germplasm is indispensable [11]. Besides abiotic stress, the deficiency of micronutrients also affects the crop production.

The crop plants are very sensitive and respond to environmental stimuli through signal perception. The plant responds accordingly for a specific environmental stimulus instigating specific physiochemical changes. These physiochemical changes or adaptations are administered by complex molecular regulatory mechanism of involving various sensors regulated by transcriptional factors/regulators. Various studies have been carried out for understanding the regulatory mechanism of plants during stress conditions. Earlier, *CIPK* genes (*OsCIPK01–OsCIPK30*) in the rice genome were studied for their transcriptional responses to various abiotic stresses [15]. The results showed that 20 *OsCIPK* genes were differentially induced by at least one of the stresses, including drought, salinity, cold, polyethylene glycol, and abscisic acid treatment. Most of the genes induced by drought or salt stress were also induced by abscisic acid treatment but not by cold. A few *CIPK* genes containing none of the reported stress-responsive *cis*-elements in their promoter regions were also induced by multiple stresses [15]. The proteins possessing A20/AN1 zinc-finger, named *SAP* gene family in rice and *Arabidopsis*, were inducible by one or the other abiotic stresses indicating that the *OsSAP* gene family is an important component of stress response in rice [16]. In addition, the role of *SAP* gene family in abiotic stress conditions was established by expression profiling under abiotic stress conditions. Seven Expansin A (*ExpA*) mRNAs were accumulated in leaves of deepwater rice, and their abundance was upregulated by submergence [17]. Similarly, the drought response in rice incites a signaling cascade through osmolyte synthesis that involves perception and translation of drought signal [18, 19].

Earlier, microarray experiments have been used for expression analysis of multiple genes during various conditions in different tissues for crop plants. The microarray experiments helped to identify the coexpressive genes during a stress condition [20–23]. Though the microarray experiments provided very useful information, the unviability of genome-wide information about the transcripts did not provide the complete information about the regulatory gene networks involved in the stress response. Nowadays, the availability of high-throughput techniques, achieved through advancement of molecular techniques, provided breakthrough in the understanding of complex regulatory gene networks and their signaling pathways involved in stress responses [24]. The techniques are comprised of whole genome transcriptome analyses, small RNA sequencing analysis (RNA-Seq), proteomic analyses, epigenetic sequencing analysis, and metabolomic analyses [25]. These high-throughput techniques use sequence-based approaches instead of hybridization-based approaches (like microarray), which require known genomic sequences, rather able to determine the transcript sequences directly from new genomes, able to map and quantify them [26, 27]. The RNA-Seq has superiority among these techniques due to its in-depth coverage of genome, global expression of transcripts, and also providing detailed information about alternative splicing and allele-specific expressions [27]. The inception of RNA-Seq technique has reformed the perception of complex and dynamic nature of the genomes, further helps to comprehensively elucidate the complex regulatory gene networks pertaining to different physiological and developmental stages of plants [28]. Currently, the various transcriptome analyses of rice genome, accomplished through RNA-Seq, during various abiotic stresses have generated enormous data. Further, these data have been able to decipher the complex regulatory gene networks in rice during various abiotic stresses which helped to understand the adaptive physiological measures taken by rice at cellular level and ascertain the development of tolerant rice varieties. Here, we are describing some of the different transcriptome studies carried out to understand the molecular responses in rice genome during various abiotic stresses.

## 2. Transcriptome data for submergence/flooding

Flooding is considered as a major threat to the rice crops, as irregular flash floods are very common in the Southeast Asia (major rice producing region), severely affecting the rice productivity [29]. Rice produces high yields, when it is grown in water-logged rice paddies. It can tolerate partial submergence as paddy rice or deepwater rice. However, it is damaged when submerged for a relatively longer period [14] due to the slow diffusion of oxygen in water fails to match the demands of respiration [30] resulting an anaerobic metabolism and energy crisis [12]. Also, in deepwater rice, energy generation through fermentative metabolism, aerenchyma development in parenchymal tissues that improves access to $O_2$, activation of ethylene promoted gibberellic acid (GA)-mediated internode elongation cause foliage to shoot up above the water surface for gas exchange and restricting growth and conserving available energy until floodwater recedes [12, 13]. Similarly, flood-tolerant rice varieties have developed the capacity to generate ATP without the presence of oxygen and/or to develop specific morphologies that improve the entrance of oxygen [31]. Moreover, the phytohormonal regulation revealed that gibberellin (GA) has negative effects on submergence tolerance, whereas paclobutrazol (PB), chemical inhibitor of GA, acted contrary to GA [32]. The transcriptome analysis between GA- and PB-treated samples and control identified 3936 differentially expressed genes largely associated with the stress response, phytohormone biosynthesis and signaling, photosynthesis, and nutrient metabolism. It was observed that the PB improved the rice survival during submergence through sustaining the photosynthesis capacity and by dropping nutrient metabolism [32].

Despite knowledge of adaptive mechanisms and regulation at the gene and protein level, our understanding of the mechanisms behind plant responses to submergence is still limited. Even in flood-intolerant species, such as *Arabidopsis thaliana*, many genes are triggered in response to flooding stress [33, 34]. The response of plants to low oxygen stress comprises complex biochemical and genetic programs that include the differential expressions of a large number of genes (**Table 1**). Gene expression is altered under low oxygen stress, and the existence of *anaerobic response elements* (*AREs*) along with their binding factors has already been reported [35]. Eventually, a *SUB1* locus and three ethylene response factors (ERFs) were identified within the locus in tolerant rice varieties (e.g., FR13A), whereas *SUB1* is a major determinant of tolerance [36]. Introduction of the *SUB1A* gene into submergence-intolerant rice variety significantly increased its flooding tolerance, thus demonstrating the importance of the *SUB1* locus for flooding tolerance [36]. Two different types of molecular mechanisms are adapted by rice ecotypes to survive under stress, *SUB1A*-mediated "quiescence strategy" [37, 38] and "escape strategy" induced by *SNORKEL1/2* [13]. The submergence response in rice consists of the differential expression of genes related to gibberellin biosynthesis, trehalose biosynthesis, anaerobic fermentation, cell wall modification, and transcription factors that include ethylene-responsive factor genes [39]. Though the regulatory mechanism in rice during submergence response has been comprehensively studied, the genome-wide gene expression as well as allelic variation among the cultivars for specific quantitative traits remained elusive. One of the studies was conducted in six rice genotypes to estimate the coleoptile elongation rates during submergence [39]. The result postulated that the coleoptile elongation was augmented by transcriptional regulation. Further, the reason for the variation in anaerobic germination was due to the allelic variation caused by the small-to-large deletions in the coding region of susceptible varieties [39].

Recently, a study on *SUB1A-1* genotypes is carried to understand the molecular mechanism pertaining to the physiological function upon desubmergence through transcriptomic analysis [29]. The results enumerated around 1400 genes that were differentially expressed to recover from the stress to preserve the plastid integrity, and the genes regulating the cell division, chromatin structure, and signaling associated with starch catabolism [29]. They also found that the rice plants recover shoot transcriptome significantly to the control state and return to homeostasis during the 24-h recovery period. It also regulated the GA-responsive starch metabolism

| Abiotic stress condition | Gene/s responsible for tolerance | Downstream key gene/s | Physiological functions |
|---|---|---|---|
| Submergence | *SUB1A* | *ERFs* regulating genes of GA-responsive starch metabolism, anaerobic fermentation, cell wall modification, JA-mediated internode elongation, and biotic responsive | Quiescence strategy to stop all physiological functions |
| | *SNORKEL1/2* | | Escape strategy to supersede water level |
| Drought | *DREBs* (*DREB1A-D/CBF1–4* and *DREB2*) | ABA-responsive genes, *LEA*, *NAC*, *DBP*, α-linolenic acid metabolic pathway genes, osmolyte biosynthesis genes, phospholipid metabolism genes; water channel protein, sugar and proline transporters, and detoxification enzyme-encoding genes; and signaling molecule-encoding genes | Stomatal closure, repression of cell growth, photosynthesis and activation of respiration and production of phytohormone ABA |
| Salt | *SOS1*, *NHX*, *HKT2*, *CAX1*, *AKT1*, *KCO1*, *TPC1*, *CLC1*, *NRT1*, *CDPK7*, *MAPK5*, *CaMBP*, *GST*, *LEA*, *V-ATPase*, *OSAP1*, and *HBP1B* | Genes related to antioxidants, transcription factors, signaling, ion and metabolic homeostasis and transporters | Imbalance in ion homeostasis of cells at plasma membrane and sequestration of vacuolar ion, and stomatal closure which causes higher leaf temperature and reserve shoot elongation |
| Cold | *CBF1*, *DREB1A*, and *DREB1B* | ABA-responsive genes, *ABF*, *NAC*, *NACRS* containing genes, *ERF922*, *WRKY25*, and *WRKY74*, gene related to signal transduction, phytohormones, antioxidant system and biotic stress | Altered chlorophyll content and fluorescence causing reduction in photosynthesis, increases content of ROS and malondialdehyde causing oxidative damage to cells |
| Cadmium (Cd) | | Cd-responsive transporters, ROS-scavenging enzymes, chelators, and metal transporter-encoding genes and many drought stress-related genes | Fatal damage to rice seedlings during their development |
| Phosphorus (P) | | RNA transport and mRNA monitoring path genes | Important for energy transfer, signal transduction, photosynthesis, and respiration |
| Manganese (Mn) | | TFs, transporters, transferase protein genes, catalytic protein encoding genes, *WRKY*, and potassium transporter-related genes, *Aux/IAA* family, and sodium transporter-related genes | Important for catalyzing the water-splitting reaction of oxygen-evolving complex in photosystem II (PSII), acts as cofactor that activates different enzymes, such as Mn-superoxide dismutase and others, to protect against oxidative stresses |
| Alkaline stress | Alkali-responsive genes | Alkaline resistant genes, TFs related to hormone signal transduction and secondary metabolite biosynthesis pathways | |

**Table 1.**
*Regulatory role of different abiotic stress-responsive genes based on RNA-Seq analysis.*

indirectly through *SUB1A* and downstream regulatory network to resume the photosynthesis [29]. Similar studies have also been carried between two contrasting deepwater growth rice cultivars [40]. The RNA-Seq analysis was conducted from different tissues, shoot base region, including basal nodes, internodes, and shoot apices of seedlings at two developmental stages. The study elucidated the possible role of jasmonic acid-mediated internode elongation and expression of biotic stress-related genes during submergence response [40].

## 3. Transcriptome data for drought stress

One of the major abiotic stresses that severely affect the rice production is drought stress. Drought stress causes a series of physiological and biochemical changes which included stomatal closure, repression of cell growth, photosynthesis, and activation of respiration along with production of the phytohormone abscisic acid (ABA) [41]. In response to the drought stress, ABA triggers stomatal closure and induces expression of stress-related genes (**Table 1**) [41]. However, some of drought-related genes were not expressed by the external ABA treatment. Therefore, the drought response is either of ABA-independent or of ABA-dependent or both inducible gene regulatory system networks [42]. These regulatory networks are the amalgamation of interaction between transcription factors and their respective promoter *cis*-elements. It was observed that the promoters of ABA-dependent genes have ABA-responsive element (*ABRE*) and, dehydration- and cold-responsive element (*C-repeat/DRE*) [42]. The transcription factors, which specifically bind to *ABRE* are known as DREBs, trigger the expression of ABA-responsive genes [43], which further encode AP2 domain-containing transcription factors regulating the stress-related genes in an ABA-independent manner [44]. The *DREB* gene family has two groups *DREB1/CBF* and *DREB2*, whereas *DREB1/CBF* consists of *DREB1A* (CBF3), *DREB1B* (CBF1), *DREB1C* (CBF2), and *DREB1D* (CBF4). However, five *DREB* homologs were identified in rice, *OsDREB1A*, *OsDREB1B*, *OsDREB1C*, *OsDREB1D*, and *OsDREB2A* [45, 46]. These gene-encoded proteins are classified into two: the first group belongs to the functional proteins included chaperones, late embryogenesis abundant (LEA) proteins, osmotin, antifreeze proteins, mRNA-binding proteins, enzymes for osmolyte biosynthesis, water channel proteins, sugar and proline transporters, and detoxification enzymes; the second group is of regulatory proteins (signal transduction and stress-responsive) including various transcription factors, protein kinases, protein phosphatases, enzymes involved in phospholipid metabolism, and other signaling molecules such as calmodulin-binding protein [22, 41]. Interestingly, it was found that many of these proteins, especially *DREBs*, are also involved in transcriptional regulation of stress-response mechanism during cold and salt stresses [46, 47].

The rice is the only crop which is grown in the waterlogged fields and it has very low water-use efficiency [48]. Therefore, it is imperative to decipher the molecular regulatory mechanism to increase the water usage efficiency of rice or the drought tolerance. Nowadays, the drought stress is continuously affecting the rice productivity due to the harsh environmental condition. The transcriptome studies proved to be the boom for researchers due to its global genomes depth and all at once allele mining among different rice genotypes. Earlier, a transcriptome analysis between drought-tolerant and drought-sensitive cultivars was carried out for the identification of novel genetic regulatory mechanisms [48]. This study suggested that the upregulation of genes related to carbon fixation, glycolysis/gluconeogenesis, and flavonoid biosynthesis, whereas the downregulation of genes associated with starch and sucrose metabolism during drought. Further, they also found the upregulation of genes associated with α-linolenic acid metabolic pathway in tolerant genotype during the stress which supported the previous findings. Consecutively, the analysis of consensus *cis*-motif among the coexpressed drought-induced genes led to the identification of novel *cis*-motifs [48]. Similar comparative studies have been carried out between tolerant and susceptible rice cultivars and in other crops to understand the regulatory mechanisms during drought [49–51]. Their result suggested that 801 transcripts differentially expressed in tolerant cultivar including the TFs NAC and DBP, and thioredoxin involved in phenylpropanoid metabolism [49].

To sustain the drought condition, the roots have a very important role. To understand the molecular regulation in rice seedling roots (4-weeks old) during drought condition, comparative RNA-Seq analysis has been carried out between wet and dry soil conditions [52]. This analysis suggested that 68% of identified genes were novel, and also found that the one of the enzymes RING box E3 ligases from ubiquitin-proteasome pathway was induced by drought. Interestingly, it was found that the *OsPhyB* represses the activity of ascorbate peroxidase and catalase-mediating reactive oxygen species (ROS) processing machinery required for drought tolerance of roots in soil condition, contrary to the previous results [52].

## 4. Transcriptome data for salt stress

Some of the abiotic stresses are complementary to each other such as the drought and salt, drought and cold stresses, etc., affecting the rice productivity. It is evident that excessive loss of water from the soil evaporation due to drought causes salt accumulation in soil. The salinity is defined as deposition of sodium chloride from natural accumulation or irrigation in soil. It causes imbalance in ion homeostasis of cells regulated by ion influx and efflux at the plasma membrane and sequestration of vacuolar ion [8]. The salt stress affects stomatal closure causing increased leaf temperature and reserved shoot elongation [53]. Studies on the salinity tolerant in rice have shown the regulation of genes related to antioxidants, transcription factors, signaling, ion and metabolic homeostasis, and transporters (**Table 1**) [54]. The identified important class of genes regulated during a salt stress in rice are *OsSOS1*, *OsNHX1* ($Na^+/H^+$ antiporters), *OsHKT2;1* ($Na^+/K^+$ symporter), *OsCAX1* ($H^+/Ca^+$ antiporter), *OsAKT1* ($K^+$ inward-rectifying channel), *OsKCO1* ($K^+$ outward-rectifying channel), *OsTPC1* ($Ca^{2+}$ permeable channel), *OsCLC1* ($Cl^-$ channel), *OsNRT1;2* (nitrate transporter), *OsCDPK7*, *OsMAPK5*, *CaMBP* (*calmodulin motif binding protein*), *GST* (*glutathione-S-transferase II*), *LEA* (*late embryogenesis abundant protein*), *V-ATPase* (*vacuolar ATP synthase 16KD proteolipid subunit*), *OSAP1* (zinc finger protein), and *HBP1B* (histone binding protein, TF) [55–63]. The salt stress response mechanism is moreover of complex physiological process pertaining to metabolic and morphological changes, which is comprehensively studied, but in rice, the molecular regulatory mechanism to salt tolerance is elusive [64]. Some of the transcriptome analyses have been completed in conjugation with the drought stress to understand the salt tolerance in rice [46, 49, 59]. Earlier, a comparative study has been carried out between salt tolerant and susceptible rice cultivars to understand the regulatory mechanisms [49]. The result suggested higher expression of bHLH and $C_2H_2$ TF family members, which might be regulating the genes associated with wax and terpenoid metabolism pathways [49]. Similarly, to understand the salinity stress, a comparative leaf transcriptome analysis at three time points on rice seedlings has been completed [65]. They identified 1375 novel genes, whereas 286 differentially expressed genes exclusively found in tolerant cultivar. They validated two genes: disease resistance response protein *206* and *TIFY10A* to understand the molecular response to salinity stress [65].

## 5. Transcriptome data for cold stress

The cold stress is defined according to the temperature affecting the plant growth and development which ranges 0–15°C (chilling stress) and <0°C (freezing stress) [66]. The tropical origin of rice makes it more susceptible to cold, critically affecting reproductive stages and grain quality leading to yield reductions [67]. The cold stress affects chlorophyll content and fluorescence causing reduction in photosynthesis, increases content of reactive oxygen species (ROS) and malondialdehyde (MDA) causing oxidative damage to cells in rice [68]. The molecular regulation of cold stress is identified in conjugation of drought stress (**Table 1**) [45]. Many stress-inducible genes are regulated via ABA-independent pathway, characteristically having a *cis* element responsible for dehydration (*DRE*) as well as low-temperature-induced expression. The low-temperature-inducible genes possess C-repeat (*CRT*) and low-temperature-responsive element (*LTRE*). The DRE-binding proteins encoding genes *CBF1*, *DREB1A*, and *DREB1B* were induced by cold stress [46]. During cold stress, ABA also accumulates and initiates the ABA signaling cascade, which regulates the ABA-responsive genes through *ABRE* and the ABRE-binding bZIP transcription factor ABF [69]. The *OsNAC* gene transduces the ABA signal through an *ABRE* in its promoter and regulates the expression of NACRS-containing genes to control cold tolerance in rice [67]. Further, to understand comprehensively the regulation of genes during cold stress, a transcriptome study is carried out between weedy and cultivated rice [70]. The analysis suggested that some typical cold stress-related genes were of basic helix-loop-helix (bHLH) gene and leucine-rich repeat (LRR) domain genes, and several genes associated with phytohormones like abscisic acid (ABA), gibberellic acid (GA), auxin, and ethylene [70]. Similarly, the wild rice, *O. longistaminata*, tolerates nonfreezing cold temperatures, is used for the identification of molecular mechanisms in response to low temperature in its shoots and rhizomes at seedling and reproductive stages using transcriptome analysis [71]. They found photosynthesis pathway-related genes were prevalent in shoots, whereas metabolic pathways and the programmed cell death process-related genes were expressed only in rhizomes. Further, they found that the TFs *CBF/DREB1*, *AP2/EREBPs*, *MYBs*, and *WRKYs* were synergistically expressed in shoots, whereas *OsERF922*, *OsNAC9*, *OsWRKY25*, *OsWRKY74*, and eight antioxidant enzymes encoding genes were expressed in rhizomes during cold stress. The *cis*-regulatory element analysis suggested the enrichment of ICE1-binding site, GATA element, and W-box in both tissues. And the highly expressed genes in shoots were associated with photosynthesis, whereas signal transduction-related genes were highly expressed in rhizomes [71].

Furthermore, a transcriptome analysis is performed in germination phase for contrasting cultivars of rice in cold stress [72], suggesting the higher expression of gene related to signal transduction, phytohormones, antioxidant system, and biotic stress during germination in cold stress [72].

## 6. Transcriptome data for trace element stress

The rice is the staple food fulfilling the dietary needs of a large population around the world. Besides dietary energy and proteins, it also contains trace elements (Li, B, Al, Cr, Mn, Fe, Co, Ni, Cu, Zn, As, Se, Sr., Mo, Cd, Ba, Pb, and Bi) in low amounts [73]. Some of these trace elements Se, Mo, Cr, Mn, Fe, Co, Cu, Zn are micronutrients that help in proper functioning of human biological systems, while nonessential heavy elements such as Pb, As, Cd, Hg are referred as toxins for consumption [73, 74]. However, the trace elements in rice are invariably increasing either due to the use of agrochemicals or irrigation with contaminated water. The deficiency or accumulation of these trace elements in soil hampers plant growth and development. On the other hand, their biofortification helps to add nutrition supplement. Henceforth, the detailed study about the effects of these trace elements on the rice is indispensable. There are many reports about trace element stresses on rice achieved through transcriptome studies (**Table 1**).

The higher concentration of heavy metal cadmium (Cd) severely hampers the rice growth. Therefore, to understand the molecular mechanism during Cd stress, transcriptome analysis has been completed by exposing rice to higher concentrations of Cd [75]. They found constitutively expressed genes were less affected by low Cd concentrations, whereas high Cd concentration causes fatal damage to rice seedlings during their development. They also found some novel Cd-responsive transporters encoding genes [75]. Previously, they found the upregulation of many genes related to ROS-scavenging enzymes, chelators, and metal transporters during Cd exposure along with upregulation of many drought stress-related genes [76].

Phosphorus (P) is an essential trace element required for proper plant growth and development where it plays an important role in energy transfer, signal transduction, photosynthesis, and respiration [77]. A comparative transcriptome study has been carried out in leaf and root tissues during phosphorus stress to elucidate their molecular mechanisms [78]. The transcriptome analysis suggested that many differentially expressed TFs and functional genes were uniquely involved in multiple regulatory pathways (including RNA transport and mRNA monitoring path) during phosphorus deficiency tolerance [78].

Manganese (Mn) is an essential trace element which plays an important role in catalyzing the water-splitting reaction of oxygen-evolving complex in photosystem II (PSII). It also acts as a cofactor that activates different enzymes, such as Mn-superoxide dismutase and others, to protect against oxidative stresses in plants [79]. However, higher Mn affects the physiological and biochemical pathways associated with plant growth and development. Therefore, to decipher the molecular mechanisms in leaves of Mn-sensitive rice exposed to high Mn stress, transcriptome analysis has been done [79]. The analysis suggested that a large number of TFs, transporters, transferase proteins, catalytic proteins encoding genes were differentially expressed having a major role in primary and secondary metabolisms. Further, it was found that the *WRKY* family and potassium transporter-related genes were significantly upregulated, whereas *Aux/IAA* family and sodium transporter-related genes were strongly downregulated [79].

## 7. Transcriptome data for other stresses

Besides common abiotic stresses, some other stresses are also studied with the help of transcriptome analysis. A transcriptome study has been carried out for alkaline stress caused by alkaline $NaHCO_3$ and $Na_2CO$ [80]. The study reported the identification of 926 differentially expressed important alkali-responsive genes including 28 alkaline-resistant genes and 74 transcription factor genes. These genes were related to hormone signal transduction and secondary metabolite biosynthesis pathways [80].

The RNA-Seq or transcriptome analysis has tremendous potential to divulge the complex molecular machinery of plant regulatory response during stress conditions. However, this large number of transcriptome data of abiotic stresses in rice has contributed significantly to rice researchers. It helped to understand complete molecular mechanism pertaining to their physiological and biochemical changes. Such data mining could be a high impact methodical source for identification of candidate gene through integration of functional genomics approach. This will also help to establish the hierarchical relationships between specific signaling components and downstream effector genes to cope up the stress conditions.

## Acknowledgements

PKD acknowledges ICAR-NASF and ICAR-NPTC for funding and support of research work at NRC on Plant Biotechnology.

## Author details

Ashutosh Kumar* and Prasanta K. Dash
ICAR-National Institute for Plant Biotechnology, PUSA, New Delhi, India

*Address all correspondence to: kr.ashutosh@yahoo.com

## References

[1] Cantrell RP, Reeves TG. The rice genome. The cereal of the world's poor takes center stage. Science. 2002;**296**(5565):53

[2] Khush GS. Origin, dispersal, cultivation and variation of rice. Plant Molecular Biology. 1997;**35**(1-2):25-34

[3] Gao J, Chao D, Lin H. Toward understanding molecular mechanisms of abiotic stress responses in rice. Rice. 2008;**1**:15

[4] Rosell CM, Marco C. Rice. In: Gluten-Free Cereal Products and Beverages. Amsterdam, Netherlands: Academic Press; 2008. p. 20

[5] Wassmann R, Jagadish SVK, Heuer S, Ismail A, Redona E, Serraj R, et al. Production: The physiological and agronomic basis for possible adaptation strategies. In: Sparks DL, editor. Advances in Agronomy. Burlington: Academic Press; 2009. p. 63

[6] Pandey P, Irulappan V, Bagavathiannan MV, Senthil-Kumar M. Impact of combined abiotic and biotic stresses on plant growth and avenues for crop improvement by exploiting physio-morphological traits. Frontiers in Plant Science. 2017;**8**:537

[7] Alqudah AM, Samarah NH, Mullen RE. Drought stress effect on crop pollination, seed set, yield and quality. In: Lichtfouse E, editor. Alternative Farming Systems, Biotechnology, Drought Stress and Ecological Fertilisation. Dordrecht: Springer; 2011. p. 20

[8] Hasegawa PM, Bressan RA, Zhu JK, Bohnert HJ. Plant cellular and molecular responses to high salinity. Annual Review of Plant Physiology and Plant Molecular Biology. 2000;**51**:463-499

[9] Shimono H, Abe A, Aoki N, Koumoto T, Sato M, Yokoi S, et al. Combining mapping of physiological quantitative trait loci and transcriptome for cold tolerance for counteracting male sterility induced by low temperatures during reproductive stage in rice. Physiologia Plantarum. 2016;**157**(2):175-192

[10] Liu CT, Wang W, Mao BG, Chu CC. Cold stress tolerance in rice: Physiological changes, molecular mechanism, and future prospects. Yi chuan = Hereditas. 2018;**40**(3):171-185

[11] Lafitte HR, Ismail A, Bennett J. Abiotic stress tolerance in rice for Asia: Progress and the future. New directions for a diverse planet. In: 4th International Crop Science Congress; Brisbane, Australia. 2004

[12] Bailey-Serres J, Voesenek LA. Flooding stress: Acclimations and genetic diversity. Annual Review of Plant Biology. 2008;**59**:313-339

[13] Hattori Y, Nagai K, Furukawa S, Song XJ, Kawano R, Sakakibara H, et al. The ethylene response factors SNORKEL1 and SNORKEL2 allow rice to adapt to deep water. Nature. 2009;**460**(7258):1026-1030

[14] Agarwal S, Grover A. Isolation and transcription profiling of low-$O_2$ stress-associated cDNA clones from the flooding-stress-tolerant FR13A rice genotype. Annals of Botany. 2005;**96**(5):831-844

[15] Xiang Y, Huang Y, Xiong L. Characterization of stress-responsive CIPK genes in rice for stress tolerance improvement. Plant Physiology. 2007;**144**(3):1416-1428

[16] Vij S, Tyagi AK. Genome-wide analysis of the stress associated protein (SAP) gene family containing A20/AN1 zinc-finger(s) in rice and their phylogenetic relationship with

*Arabidopsis*. Molecular Genetics and Genomics. 2006;**276**(6):565-575

[17] Lee Y, Kende H. Expression of alpha-expansin and expansin-like genes in Deepwater rice. Plant Physiology. 2002;**130**(3):1396-1405

[18] Dash PK, Rai R, Rai V, Pasupalak S. Drought induced signaling in rice: Delineating canonical and non-canonical pathways. Frontiers in Chemistry. 2018;**6**:264

[19] Shivaraj SM, Deshmukh RK, Rai R, Belanger R, Agrawal PK, Dash PK. Genome-wide identification, characterization, and expression profile of aquaporin gene family in flax (*Linum usitatissimum*). Scientific Reports. 2017;7:46137

[20] Lasanthi-Kudahettige R, Magneschi L, Loreti E, Gonzali S, Licausi F, Novi G, et al. Transcript profiling of the anoxic rice coleoptile. Plant Physiology. 2007;**144**(1):218-231

[21] Lee WP, Tzou WS. Computational methods for discovering gene networks from expression data. Briefings in Bioinformatics. 2009;**10**(4):408-423

[22] Rabbani MA, Maruyama K, Abe H, Khan MA, Katsura K, Ito Y, et al. Monitoring expression profiles of rice genes under cold, drought, and high-salinity stresses and abscisic acid application using cDNA microarray and RNA gel-blot analyses. Plant Physiology. 2003;**133**(4):1755-1767

[23] Dash PK, Cao Y, Jailani AK, Gupta P, Venglat P, Xiang D, et al. Genome-wide analysis of drought induced gene expression changes in flax (*Linum usitatissimum*). GM Crops & Food. 2014;**5**(2):106-119

[24] Grennan AK. Abiotic stress in rice. An "omic" approach. Plant Physiology. 2006;**140**(4):1139-1141

[25] Sana TR, Fischer S, Wohlgemuth G, Katrekar A, Jung KH, Ronald PC, et al. Metabolomic and transcriptomic analysis of the rice response to the bacterial blight pathogen *Xanthomonas oryzae* pv. oryzae. Metabolomics: Official Journal of the Metabolomic Society. 2010;**6**(3):451-465

[26] Wang Z, Gerstein M, Snyder M. RNA-Seq: A revolutionary tool for transcriptomics. Nature Reviews Genetics. 2009;**10**(1):57-63

[27] Kukurba KR, Montgomery SB. RNA sequencing and analysis. Cold Spring Harbor Protocols. 2015;**2015**(11):951-969

[28] Dash PK, Rai R, Mahato AK, Gaikwad K, Singh NK. Transcriptome landscape at different developmental stages of a drought tolerant cultivar of flax (*Linum usitatissimum*). Frontiers in Chemistry. 2017;**5**:82

[29] Locke AM, Barding GA Jr, Sathnur S, Larive CK, Bailey-Serres J. Rice SUB1A constrains remodelling of the transcriptome and metabolome during submergence to facilitate post-submergence recovery. Plant, Cell & Environment. 2018;**41**(4):721-736

[30] Mohanty B, Krishnan SP, Swarup S, Bajic VB. Detection and preliminary analysis of motifs in promoters of anaerobically induced genes of different plant species. Annals of Botany. 2005;**96**(4):669-681

[31] Voesenek LA, Colmer TD, Pierik R, Millenaar FF, Peeters AJ. How plants cope with complete submergence. The New Phytologist. 2006;**170**(2):213-226

[32] Xiang J, Wu H, Zhang Y, Zhang Y, Wang Y, Li Z, et al. Transcriptomic analysis of gibberellin- and paclobutrazol-treated rice seedlings under submergence. International Journal of Molecular Sciences. 2017;**18**(10):1-16

[33] Branco-Price C, Kawaguchi R, Ferreira RB, Bailey-Serres J. Genome-wide analysis of transcript abundance and translation in *Arabidopsis* seedlings subjected to oxygen deprivation. Annals of Botany. 2005;**96**(4):647-660

[34] Gonzali S, Loreti E, Novi G, Poggi A, Alpi A, Perata P. The use of microarrays to study the anaerobic response in *Arabidopsis*. Annals of Botany. 2005;**96**(4):661-668

[35] Klok EJ, Wilson IW, Wilson D, Chapman SC, Ewing RM, Somerville SC, et al. Expression profile analysis of the low-oxygen response in *Arabidopsis* root cultures. The Plant Cell. 2002;**14**(10):2481-2494

[36] Xu K, Xu X, Fukao T, Canlas P, Maghirang-Rodriguez R, Heuer S, et al. Sub1A is an ethylene-response-factor-like gene that confers submergence tolerance to rice. Nature. 2006;**442**(7103):705-708

[37] Voesenek LA, Bailey-Serres J. Flood adaptive traits and processes: An overview. The New Phytologist. 2015;**206**(1):57-73

[38] Bailey-Serres J, Voesenek LA. Life in the balance: A signaling network controlling survival of flooding. Current Opinion in Plant Biology. 2010;**13**(5):489-494

[39] Hsu SK, Tung CW. RNA-Seq analysis of diverse Rice genotypes to identify the genes controlling coleoptile growth during submerged germination. Frontiers in Plant Science. 2017;**8**:762

[40] Minami A, Yano K, Gamuyao R, Nagai K, Kuroha T, Ayano M, et al. Time-course transcriptomics analysis reveals key responses of submerged deepwater rice to flooding. Plant Physiology. 2018;**176**(4):3081-3102

[41] Shinozaki K, Yamaguchi-Shinozaki K. Gene networks involved in drought stress response and tolerance. Journal of Experimental Botany. 2007;**58**(2):221-227

[42] Yamaguchi-Shinozaki K, Shinozaki K. Organization of cis-acting regulatory elements in osmotic- and cold-stress-responsive promoters. Trends in Plant Science. 2005;**10**(2):88-94

[43] Stockinger EJ, Gilmour SJ, Thomashow MF. *Arabidopsis thaliana* CBF1 encodes an AP2 domain-containing transcriptional activator that binds to the C-repeat/DRE, a cis-acting DNA regulatory element that stimulates transcription in response to low temperature and water deficit. Proceedings of the National Academy of Sciences of the United States of America. 1997;**94**(3):1035-1040

[44] Shinozaki K, Yamaguchi-Shinozaki K. Molecular responses to dehydration and low temperature: Differences and cross-talk between two stress signaling pathways. Current Opinion in Plant Biology. 2000;**3**(3):217-223

[45] Sakuma Y, Liu Q, Dubouzet JG, Abe H, Shinozaki K, Yamaguchi-Shinozaki K. DNA-binding specificity of the ERF/AP2 domain of *Arabidopsis* DREBs, transcription factors involved in dehydration- and cold-inducible gene expression. Biochemical and Biophysical Research Communications. 2002;**290**(3):998-1009

[46] Dubouzet JG, Sakuma Y, Ito Y, Kasuga M, Dubouzet EG, Miura S, et al. OsDREB genes in rice, *Oryza sativa* L., encode transcription activators that function in drought-, high-salt- and cold-responsive gene expression. The Plant Journal: For Cell and Molecular Biology. 2003;**33**(4):751-763

[47] Chen JQ, Meng XP, Zhang Y, Xia M, Wang XP. Over-expression of OsDREB genes lead to enhanced drought tolerance in rice. Biotechnology Letters. 2008;**30**(12):2191-2198

[48] Lenka SK, Katiyar A, Chinnusamy V, Bansal KC. Comparative analysis of drought-responsive transcriptome in Indica rice genotypes with contrasting drought tolerance. Plant Biotechnology Journal. 2011;**9**(3):315-327

[49] Shankar R, Bhattacharjee A, Jain M. Transcriptome analysis in different rice cultivars provides novel insights into desiccation and salinity stress responses. Scientific Reports. 2016;**6**:23719

[50] Gupta P, Dash PK. Molecular details of secretory phospholipase A2 from flax (*Linum usitatissimum* L.) provide insight into its structure and function. Scientific Reports. 2017;**7**(1):11080

[51] Gupta P, Saini R, Dash PK. Origin and evolution of group XI secretory phospholipase A2 from flax (*Linum usitatissimum*) based on phylogenetic analysis of conserved domains. 3 Biotech. 2017;**7**(3):216

[52] Yoo YH, Nalini Chandran AK, Park JC, Gho YS, Lee SW, An G, et al. OsPhyB-mediating novel regulatory pathway for drought tolerance in Rice root identified by a global RNA-Seq transcriptome analysis of rice genes in response to water deficiencies. Frontiers in Plant Science. 2017;**8**:580

[53] Rajendran K, Tester M, Roy SJ. Quantifying the three main components of salinity tolerance in cereals. Plant, Cell & Environment. 2009;**32**(3):237-249

[54] Das P, Nutan KK, Singla-Pareek SL, Pareek A. Understanding salinity responses and adopting 'omics-based' approaches to generate salinity tolerant cultivars of rice. Frontiers in Plant Science. 2015;**6**:712

[55] Kumar K, Kumar M, Kim SR, Ryu H, Cho YG. Insights into genomics of salt stress response in rice. Rice (NY). 2013;**6**(1):27

[56] Mishra S, Singh B, Panda K, Singh BP, Singh N, Misra P, et al. Association of SNP haplotypes of HKT family genes with salt tolerance in Indian wild Rice germplasm. Rice (NY). 2016;**9**(1):15

[57] Yang T, Zhang S, Hu Y, Wu F, Hu Q, Chen G, et al. The role of a potassium transporter OsHAK5 in potassium acquisition and transport from roots to shoots in rice at low potassium supply levels. Plant Physiology. 2014;**166**(2):945-959

[58] Kurusu T, Hamada H, Koyano T, Kuchitsu K. Intracellular localization and physiological function of a rice Ca(2)(+)-permeable channel OsTPC1. Plant Signaling & Behavior. 2012;**7**(11):1428-1430

[59] Golldack D, Quigley F, Michalowski CB, Kamasani UR, Bohnert HJ. Salinity stress-tolerant and -sensitive rice (*Oryza sativa* L.) regulate AKT1-type potassium channel transcripts differently. Plant Molecular Biology. 2003;**51**(1):71-81

[60] Wang H, Zhang M, Guo R, Shi D, Liu B, Lin X, et al. Effects of salt stress on ion balance and nitrogen metabolism of old and young leaves in rice (*Oryza sativa* L.). BMC Plant Biology. 2012;**12**:194

[61] Xiong L, Yang Y. Disease resistance and abiotic stress tolerance in rice are inversely modulated by an abscisic acid-inducible mitogen-activated protein kinase. The Plant Cell. 2003;**15**(3):745-759

[62] Saijo Y, Hata S, Kyozuka J, Shimamoto K, Izui K. Over-expression of a single $Ca^{2+}$-dependent protein kinase confers both cold and salt/drought tolerance on rice plants. The Plant Journal: For Cell and Molecular Biology. 2000;**23**(3):319-327

[63] Kumari S, Sabharwal VP, Kushwaha HR, Sopory SK, Singla-Pareek SL, Pareek A. Transcriptome map for seedling stage specific salinity stress

response indicates a specific set of genes as candidate for saline tolerance in *Oryza sativa* L. Functional & Integrative Genomics. 2009;**9**(1):109-123

[64] Rahman MA, Thomson MJ, Shah EAM, de Ocampo M, Egdane J, Ismail AM. Exploring novel genetic sources of salinity tolerance in rice through molecular and physiological characterization. Annals of Botany. 2016;**117**(6):1083-1097

[65] Wang J, Zhu J, Zhang Y, Fan F, Li W, Wang F, et al. Comparative transcriptome analysis reveals molecular response to salinity stress of salt-tolerant and sensitive genotypes of indica rice at seedling stage. Scientific Reports. 2018;**8**(1):2085

[66] Zhu J, Dong CH, Zhu JK. Interplay between cold-responsive gene regulation, metabolism and RNA processing during plant cold acclimation. Current Opinion in Plant Biology. 2007;**10**(3):290-295

[67] Zhang Q, Chen Q, Wang S, Hong Y, Wang Z. Rice and cold stress: Methods for its evaluation and summary of cold tolerance-related quantitative trait loci. Rice (NY). 2014;**7**(1):24

[68] Xie G, Kato H, Sasaki K, Imai R. A cold-induced thioredoxin h of rice, OsTrx23, negatively regulates kinase activities of OsMPK3 and OsMPK6 in vitro. FEBS Letters. 2009;**583**(17):2734-2738

[69] Hossain MA, Cho JI, Han M, Ahn CH, Jeon JS, An G, et al. The ABRE-binding bZIP transcription factor OsABF2 is a positive regulator of abiotic stress and ABA signaling in rice. Journal of Plant Physiology. 2010;**167**(17):1512-1520

[70] Guan S, Xu Q, Ma D, Zhang W, Xu Z, Zhao M, et al. Transcriptomics profiling in response to cold stress in cultivated rice and weedy rice. Gene. 2019;**685**:96-105

[71] Zhang T, Huang L, Wang Y, Wang W, Zhao X, Zhang S, et al. Differential transcriptome profiling of chilling stress response between shoots and rhizomes of *Oryza longistaminata* using RNA sequencing. PLoS One. 2017;**12**(11):e0188625

[72] da Maia LC, Cadore PRB, Benitez LC, Danielowski R, Braga EJB, Fagundes PRR, et al. Transcriptome profiling of rice seedlings under cold stress. Functional Plant Biology. 2016;**44**(4):419-429

[73] Diyabalanage S, Navarathna T, Abeysundara HT, Rajapakse S, Chandrajith R. Trace elements in native and improved paddy rice from different climatic regions of Sri Lanka: Implications for public health. Springerplus. 2016;**5**(1):1864

[74] Sebastian A, Prasad MNV. Trace element management in rice. Agronomy. 2015;**5**:30

[75] Oono Y, Yazawa T, Kanamori H, Sasaki H, Mori S, Handa H, et al. Genome-wide transcriptome analysis of cadmium stress in rice. BioMed Research International. 2016;**2016**:9739505

[76] Oono Y, Yazawa T, Kawahara Y, Kanamori H, Kobayashi F, Sasaki H, et al. Genome-wide transcriptome analysis reveals that cadmium stress signaling controls the expression of genes in drought stress signal pathways in rice. PLoS One. 2014;**9**(5):e96946

[77] Abel S, Ticconi CA, Delatorre CA. Phosphate sensing in higher plants. Physiologia Plantarum. 2002;**115**(1):1-8

[78] Deng QW, Luo XD, Chen YL, Zhou Y, Zhang FT, Hu BL, et al. Transcriptome analysis of phosphorus stress responsiveness in the seedlings of Dongxiang wild rice (*Oryza rufipogon* Griff.). Biological Research. 2018;**51**(1):7

[79] Li P, Song A, Li Z, Fan F, Liang Y. Transcriptome analysis in leaves of rice (*Oryza sativa*) under high manganese stress. Biologia. 2017;**72**(4):9

[80] Li N, Liu H, Sun J, Zheng H, Wang J, Yang L, et al. Transcriptome analysis of two contrasting rice cultivars during alkaline stress. Scientific Reports. 2018;**8**(1):9586

Chapter 6

# Revealing the Symmetry of Conifer Transcriptomes through Triplet Statistics

*Sadovsky Michael, Putintseva Yulia, Biryukov Vladislav and Senashova Maria*

## Abstract

The novel powerful technique is used for a study of combinatorial and statistical properties of transcriptome sequences. The main approach stands on the study of distribution of nucleotide triplet frequency dictionaries obtained from the conversion of transcriptome sequences. The distribution is revealed through PCA presentation and elastic map technique. The transcriptomic data of Siberian larch (*Larix sibirica* Ledeb.) and Siberian pine (*Pinus sibirica* Du Tour) were studied. The transcriptomes exhibit unusual symmetries. The octahedral structure exhibiting rotational symmetry in transcriptome contig distribution was found for *L. sibirica*, while mirror symmetry was found for *P. sibirica*. The octahedron structure seems to be universal for plants.

**Keywords:** Chargaff's parity, order, structuredness, mirror symmetry, rotational symmetry

## 1. Introduction

A discovery of an order and new structures in genetic entities is an up-to-date scientific problem. Indeed, the amount of primary genomic data shows the daily growth for billions of megabases. The symbol sequences from four-letter alphabet $= \{A, C, G, T\}$ (with few variations in some nucleotide sequences; say, U substitutes T in RNAs).

We studied an order and structuredness over a set of sequences representing the transcriptome of Siberian larch (*Larix sibirica* Ledeb.) and Siberian pine (*Pinus sibirica* Du Tour), also known as Siberian cedar. Transcriptome represents sequences of expressed genes and corresponds to the mRNA molecule isolated from biological cells or tissues. Obviously, whether a transcriptome exhibits structuredness or not heavily depends on the concept of a structuredness to be revealed and analyzed. One may face a huge number of patterns claimed to be structural units; a number of papers report on newly discovered structures in genomes [1].

There are two approaches to discuss structuredness in a set of symbol sequences (transcriptome nucleotide sequences, in our case). The first implies that one seeks for inhomogeneities in the mutual distribution of the sequences form the ensemble under consideration. Of course, to do it, one must introduce a metrics to measure the difference between any two sequences; there are various ways to do it [2–4]. An alignment might be such a measure [5, 6] (see also much more prominent approach presented in [7, 8]). Alternatively, the second approach implies the search for inhomogeneities within a sequence, e.g., through the comparison of the formally identified fragments of a sequence.

Regardless the specific approach to seek for structuredness, one must introduce a way to measure the difference between the objects to be analyzed. Alignment [9–11] is the most widespread approach here. An alternative idea to search a structure and order in symbol sequences is to transform them into frequency dictionary [12–15]. A frequency dictionary could be defined in various ways, but basically it is a list of all the strings of a given length accompanied with a frequency of each string (a detailed description is given below). A transformation of a symbol sequence into a frequency dictionary provides a mapping of a set of sequences into a metric space. Hence, one may apply all the tools for analysis.

As soon, as a structure in ensemble of sequences, or over a sequence is defined, the question arises toward the properties of those structures. Probably, symmetry of such structures is the most fundamental and basic one. Again, there could be various notions of the symmetry. The first concept of the symmetry aims to figure out structures that seem to remain similar, when some simple transformations in a proper space are provided. First of all, a rotational symmetry of a cluster structure [3, 4] or mirror symmetry [16, 17] must be mentioned here.

Few words should be said toward the symmetry. Here we shall consider two notions of that issue. The first is a well-known rotational, mirror, or similar symmetry observed in the distribution of the contigs converted into triplet frequency dictionary as they are distributed in the relevant Euclidean space (where the triplets are the coordinates). The second issue is measured through the proximity (or deviation) to Chargaff's parity rules, to be observed for various entities, both natural (these are contigs) and artificial (kernels or arithmetic means of the frequency of identical triplets counted over an ensemble of contigs).

## 2. Material and methods

### 2.1 Transcriptome nucleotide sequence data

The transcriptomes of Siberian larch and Siberian pine were originally sequenced under the project on the whole genome sequencing of Siberian larch [18, 19]. The sequence data of *L. sibirica* and *P. sibirica* were obtained using Illumina MiSeq sequencer at the Laboratory of Forest Genomics of the Siberian Federal University. The RNA was isolated from buds [19].

#### *2.1.1 L. sibirica bud transcriptome*

For the purposes of our study, we have selected the bud transcriptome of *L. sibirica*; we have taken into consideration the transcripts longer than 600 bp. The longest one in the transcriptome is as long as 10,795 bp, with average length $\langle L \rangle =$ 1243.4 bp and standard deviation $\sigma_{\langle L \rangle} = 717.9$ bp.

The total number of sequences in the transcriptome is 12,353 transcripts. The histograms of the distribution of the transcriptome sequence entries over their length are presented in **Figure 1**. Evidently, the distribution resembles Poisson distribution quite strongly. There are 7573 transcripts in the transcriptome bearing a single CDS (maybe in various directions). Four thousand thirty-eight transcripts

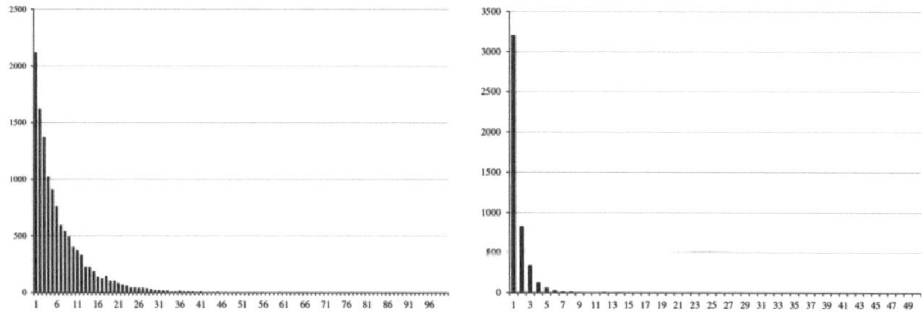

**Figure 1.**
*Distribution of L. sibirica contigs over the length (left) and P. sibirica (right).*

| # | 2 | 3 | 4 | 5 | 6 | 7 | 8 | 20 |
|---|---|---|---|---|---|---|---|---|
| *L. sibirica* | 3049 | 738 | 175 | 61 | 8 | 2 | 2 | 1 |
| *P. sibirica* | 962 | 226 | 41 | 14 | 3 | — | — | — |

*#—number of CDS in a transcript.*

**Table 1.**
*Distribution of number of CDS per transcript.*

have two or more CDS in them; the distribution of number of CDS in transcripts is shown in **Table 1**. Finally, in 742 transcripts no CDS have been found.

### 2.1.2 *P. sibirica* bud transcriptome

We used bud transcriptome from *Pinus sibirica* obtained from witch's broom (i.e., morphologically different part of a tree). It might be considered as a disease. Again, we have selected the transcripts longer that 600 bp that yields 4675 entries in the transcriptome, 3003 among them have a single CDS.

There are as many as 426 transcripts with no CDS detected in them. Surprisingly, there are no transcripts in the transcriptome with CDS belonging to both strands, simultaneously. The distribution of number of CDS found in a transcript is shown in **Table 1**. On the contrary to *L. sibirica* transcriptome, *P. sibirica* transcriptome contains no transcript without CDS

## 2.2 Triplet frequency dictionary

Triplet frequency dictionary $W_{(3,\,t)}$ is the list of all 64 triplets found within a sequence under consideration, where each entry (triplet) $\omega$ is assigned with the frequency $f_\omega$ of the triplet $\omega$. The reading frame move $t$ could be chosen arbitrary and depends on the specific problem to be solved. Everywhere further we use $t = 1$ or $t = 3$; for $t = 1$ we use the notation of $W_3$, unless it makes a confusion.

A frequency dictionary $W_{(3,\,t)}$ unambiguously maps a sequence into a point in 64-dimensional metric space. Strongly speaking, $W_{(3,\,t)}$ with $t>1$ maps a subsequence into the point of the metric space, not the sequence entirely; further we shall discuss this point in more detail. Next, the dimension of the space is 63, not 64; this fact follows from the linear constraint:

$$\sum_{\omega=\mathrm{AAA}}^{\mathrm{TTT}} f_\omega = 1. \tag{1}$$

This constraint allows to exclude any triplet from the analysis, thus changing 64-dimensional space for 63-dimensional, where all variables are linearly independent [20].

Formally speaking, any triplet could be excluded. Practically, one must eliminate the triplet with the least standard deviation figure determined over the set of frequencies under consideration. Indeed, suppose a triplet $\omega^*$ yields the standard deviation equal to zero, as determined over a set of dictionaries, it means, all dictionaries in the set have the same frequency, for this triplet: $f^j_{\omega^*} = const, \forall j$ (here $j$ enlists the dictionaries in the set). Such invariance makes the dictionaries (and the sequences standing behind) indistinguishable, from the point of view of the triplet. The choice of a triplet with minimal standard deviation for the exclusion provides the elimination of the variable contributing least of all in distinguishability of the entities.

### 2.2.1 Metric choice

The list of triplets accompanied with the frequency of each entry makes frequency dictionary $W_{(3,t)}$; let $t = 1$, at the moment. Hence, a dictionary is a point in metric space; obviously, one may define metrics in a number of ways, in such space. For the purposes of further analysis, we use the Euclidean metrics:

$$\rho\left(W_3^{[i]}, W_3^{[j]}\right) = \sqrt{\sum_{\omega=\mathrm{AAA}}^{\mathrm{TTT}} \left(f_\omega^{[j]} - f_\omega^{[i]}\right)^2}. \qquad (2)$$

Some other metrics might be used, as well. Here $i$ and $j$ index two different dictionaries (sequences, respectively).

## 2.3 Chargaff's imparity index

To begin with, we bring to mind the well-known complementarity pattern established by E. Chargaff in 1952 [21, 22]; it consists in a strong equality of A's and T's numbers (C's and G's numbers, respectively) counted over DNA molecule. Of course, some minor violations may take place due to mutations; meanwhile the accuracy of this equality is very high. This fact is also known as the first Chargaff's parity rule.

The second Chargaff's parity rule stipulates that

$$n_\mathrm{A} \approx n_\mathrm{T} \quad \text{and} \quad n_\mathrm{C} \approx n_\mathrm{G}, \qquad (3)$$

if counted within a single strand. The accuracy of (3) is rather high but varies for different taxa.

Surprisingly, similar to (3) relations are observed for oligonucleotides counted over a single stand. Let us now introduce some rigorous definitions and notions.

Definition 1. Consider a string $\omega = \nu_1\nu_2 \ldots \nu_{q-1}\nu_q$ be an oligonucleotide of the length $q$, where $\nu_j$ is nucleotide occupying the $j$-th position. *Palindrome* is the word $\omega^* = \nu_1^*\nu_2^* \ldots \nu_{q-1}^*\nu_q^*$ read equally in the opposite direction: $\nu_j = \nu_{q-j}^*$.

Definition 2. Two strings $\omega$ and $\overline{\omega}$ make the complementary palindrome, if they are read equally in the opposite directions, with respect to Chargaff's complementarity rule:

$$\mathrm{A} \Leftrightarrow \mathrm{T} \qquad \mathrm{C} \Leftrightarrow \mathrm{G}.$$

Hence, $\forall j,\ 1 \le j \le q\ \nu_j \mapsto \nu^*_{q-j+1}$. Here are some examples of complementary palindromes:

$$\text{ACT} \Leftrightarrow \text{AGT}, \quad \text{ACTGG} \Leftrightarrow \text{CCAGT}, \quad \text{ACGT} \Leftrightarrow \text{ACGT}.$$

So, the generalized second Chargaff's rule stipulates equality (or proximity, to be exact) of frequencies of two strings comprising complementary palindrome [23–33]. Surely, one hardly could expect to get the absolute equality of the frequencies of any two strings comprising complementary palindrome. There is a number of reasons standing behind the violation of such absolute equality; they range from purely combinatorial [25–27, 34] and/or finite sampling effect to biological peculiarities [24, 28, 30, 33].

To reveal the difference between genetic entities or biological objects, one must introduce a measure of the violation of the generalized second Chargaff's rule; one may do it in various ways; we use the discrepancy index:

$$\mu\left(W_q^{[i]}, W_q^{[j]}\right) = 4^{-q} \cdot \sqrt{\sum_{\omega \in \Omega} \left(f_\omega - f_{\overline{\omega}}\right)^2}. \tag{4}$$

Here $\Omega$ is the set of strings of the length $q$ observed in two sequences ($i$ and $j$, respectively), $\omega$ enlists all the strings, and $\overline{\omega}$ is the string complementary palindromic to $\omega$. Normalization factor $4^{-q}$ is introduced to equalize the figures (4) observed for various $q$.

The index (4) measures the discrepancy between two dictionaries ($W_q^{[i]}$ and $W_q^{[j]}$). Meanwhile, this index could be applied for a single frequency dictionary $W_q$:

$$\mu^\star\left(W_q\right) = 2 \cdot 4^{-q} \cdot \sqrt{\sum_{\omega \in \Omega^\star} \left(f_\omega - f_{\omega^\star}\right)^2}. \tag{5}$$

Here the complementary palindromic couples are combined from the strings belonging to the same frequency dictionary $W_q$.

The discrepancy measure (4) looks like Euclidean distance, while it is not. More exactly, it could be considered as a metrics in Euclidean space. To do it, one must reconsider a point in a couple, changing it for the dual one that is a complementary palindrome.

The inner discrepancy measure (5) definitely is not a distance, since it characterizes a single object, not a couple.

### 2.4 $W_{(3,\,3)}$ and $W_3$ dictionaries

This is a very common fact that a genome comprises coding and noncoding regions. Basically, they differ in the statistical properties manifested in triplet frequency dictionaries. One might detect some minor difference in $W_3$ composition developed for coding vs. noncoding regions. Significantly greater difference between these two types of genome parts is observed for $W_{(3,\,3)}$ dictionaries [2–4].

Dictionary $W_3$ is uniformly defined, for any sequence. The situation differs for $W_{(3,\,3)}$ dictionaries. Consider a sequence $\mathfrak{L}$ of the length $N$. Starting to cover the sequence with the frames of the length 3 moving along the sequence with the step 3, one may get three different dictionaries, in dependence to the location of the start point. The starts may be located at the first nucleotide of a sequence, at the second nucleotide, and at the third nucleotide; thus, three different triplet frequency dictionaries $W_{(3,\,3)}$ could be obtained.

The key difference between coding and noncoding regions consists in the deviations between these three dictionaries. In other words, let the sequence $\mathfrak{L}$ falls entirely into a noncoding region of a genome. One may develop three triplet frequency dictionaries $W^{[j]}_{(3,3)}$, $0 \le j \le 2$ corresponding to three positions of the reading frame shift (these are 0, 1, and 2). The key issue is that these three dictionaries:

1. Differ significantly if developed for coding and noncoding regions.

2. Differ each other, if developed for a coding region.

3. Differ between them negligibly, if developed for a noncoding region.

In other words, consider a set $\hat{W}^{[j]}_{(3,3)}$, $0 \le j \le 2$ developed over a noncoding region and a set $\tilde{W}^{[j]}_{(3,3)}$, $0 \le j \le 2$ developed over a coding region. Then, $\forall j$ the difference between $\hat{W}^{[j]}_{(3,3)}$ is rather small, when expressed in any way (as Euclidean distance, entropy, mutual entropy, etc.; see also [7, 8]), but the difference between $\tilde{W}^{[j]}_{(3,3)}$ is significantly greater. Besides, $\forall i, j$ the difference between $\tilde{W}^{[i]}_{(3,3)}$ and $\hat{W}^{[j]}_{(3,3)}$ manifests apparently. These deviations in statistical properties of such triplet frequency stand behind the *Hidden Markov Model* methodology [35, 36].

We shall explore structuredness in transcriptomes through the analysis of those triplet dictionaries developed over the individual transcripts.

## 2.5 Relative phase

To reveal the inner structuredness of a (bacterial) genome, Gorban and coauthors have introduced special construction that might be called *tiling* [2–4]. The idea was to cover a genome (considered as a symbol sequence from ) with a set of overlapping and ordered windows called tiles. All tiles are of the same length $L$ ($L = 603$ in [2–4, 16, 17]); the tiles are located along a sequence with the permanent step $P$. In the papers mentioned above, $P = 11$, and the choice of the specific figures of $L$ and $P$ is determined by the specific task of a research.

A subsequence identified by a specific tile is then converted into frequency dictionary $W_{(3,3)}$, and the inner structuredness of a genome is represented through the distribution of the points corresponding to tiles, in 64-dimensional (or 63-dimensional) metric space.

This structuredness is basically determined by the so-called *relative phase* of a tile. It may:

1. Fall completely into a coding region.

2. Fall completely outside a coding region.

3. Contain a border between coding and noncoding regions.

In any chance, the relative phase indicates whether the start of a tile coincides with a start of a coding region or not. There are following combinations determining the relative phase index:

1. Start of a coding region coincides to the start of a tile. In this case relative phase $\delta = 0$.

2. Start of a coding region does not coincide to the start of a tile, and the reminder of the division of the distance (expressed in number of nucleotides) from the start of the tile, and the start of coding region is 1. Then $\delta = 1$ in this case.

3. Finally, the start of a coding region falling inside the tile does not coincide to the start of a tile, and the remainder is 2. Then $\delta = 2$ in this case.

For any tile covering a noncoding region, $\delta = 4$, by definition.

It should be stressed that genes (or coding regions) may take place in opposite strands; in such capacity, the relative phase index must be defined for leading strand and lagging one, separately, where the remainder of the division must be determined for the difference between the last symbol of a tile and the last nucleotide of a gene annotated in a sequence as located in the lagging strand. Thus, seven figures of the relative phase index $\delta$ are possible: $F_0$, $F_1$, and $F_2$ for the tiles containing coding regions from the leading strand; $B_0$, $B_1$, and $B_2$ for the tiles containing coding regions from the lagging strand; and, finally, $J$ labeling the tiles covering noncoding regions, only.

For genome tiling (see [2–4, 16, 17]), the labeling of tiles with the relative phase index is based on genome annotation.

### 2.5.1 Transcriptome relative phase

The situation is slightly different for transcriptome (and the transcriptomes of *L. sibirica* Ledeb. and *P. sibirica* Du Tour, specifically). First of all, we did not develop any tiling, for transcripts; reciprocally, the transcripts themselves have been considered as tiles. It means that each transcript was converted into $W_{(3,\,3)}$ frequency dictionary as a whole, with no dissection into tiles.

Each frequency dictionary corresponding to a specific transcript was labeled with relative phase index; the labeling procedure was pretty close to that one described above, with few exceptions. We used `TransDecoder`™ software to find the start of a coding region within a transcript, as well as the strand location of CDS.

The relative phase index for transcripts containing a single CDS was determined in completely the same way, as described above. The transcripts bearing no CDS, if any, have been labeled with index $J$. Finally, the problem arose from the transcripts bearing several CDS: obviously, a relative phase index is defined ambiguously for such transcripts. In such capacity, we labeled the transcripts with multiple CDS with special figure $M$ of the relative phase index.

Finally, we have calculated the standard deviation for each triplet, over the entire set of transcripts; that is CGT with $\sigma_{\mathrm{CGT}} = 0.005586$, so we excluded this triplet from the set of variables to cluster the transcripts. Reciprocally, the triplet with $\sigma_{\mathrm{TGA}} = 0.014924$ yields the maximal figure of the standard deviation.

Similar figures determined for *P. sibirica* are $\sigma_{\mathrm{GCG}} = 0.005658$ and $\sigma_{\mathrm{TGA}} = 0.014936$, correspondingly; the former stands for the minimal standard deviation figure, and the latter stands for the maximal one. Hence, in cedar transcriptome, we have excluded GCG triplet. Remarkably, the triplets with the largest standard deviation figures coincide, for these two genetic entities.

## 3. Results

Previously, seven cluster symmetric patterns have been reported [2–4], in bacterial genomes. Later, similar (but not equivalent) structures were found in chloroplast genomes [16, 17]. First of all, the tiles corresponding to specific relative phase tend to aggregate into clusters apparently seen in the projection into three principal components with the largest eigenvalues. The points corresponding to specific strand (either leading or a lagging one) perform a triangle, in the frequency space; the points corresponding to noncoding regions tend to gather into a ball-like structure located in the central part of the pattern.

The patterns described in [2–4, 16, 17] are provided by the interplay of two triangles and the central ball. The triangles comprise the points corresponding to specific strand. There are two basic symmetries found in these triangles: the former is a shift (rotational) symmetry peculiar for bacterial genomes [2–4], and the latter is mirror symmetry peculiar for chloroplasts [16, 17]. The ball comprise the points corresponding to the tiles with noncoding regions inside (chloroplast genomes have one more cluster called *tail*; meanwhile, it is not important at the moment).

Whether a pattern would have four or seven clusters depends on GC content of a genome, for bacteria [2–4]. This figure almost completely determines the mutual location of the planes comprising the triangles formed by the clusters belonging to the same strand. There are some exclusions from this rule, for cyanobacteria. Chloroplasts exhibit mirror symmetry in the strand-specific triangles, so they always have a four-beam structure, where the triangles occupy the same plane with obligatory coincidence of $F_2$ and $B_2$ phases [16, 17].

### 3.1 Phase index coloring agreement

To make the presentation of results clearer, let us fix the color and label mark usage for transcripts to be shown in figures everywhere further. Indeed, we should distinguish eight different phases in the figures: $F_0$, $B_0$, $F_1$, $B_1$, $F_2$, $B_2$, *mult*, and *noCDS*.

To do that, we shall use the following labels: all phases of $F_0$ through $F_2$ of transcripts from the leading strand are marked with triangles; all phases of $B_0$ through $B_2$ of transcripts from the lagging strand are marked with diamonds; *mult* transcripts are marked with teal squares; finally, the transcripts where no CDS have been found are labeled with brown circles.

Besides, the relative phases of single CDS transcripts are colored in the following manner: $F_0$ is purple triangle, $F_1$ is lime triangle, and $F_2$ is yellow triangle; reciprocally, $B_0$ is magenta diamond, $B_1$ is azure diamond, and $B_2$ is sand diamond.

We should say few words concerning the distribution of the transcripts with several CDS detected in them. For both transcriptomes, the distribution of such transcripts in the 63-dimensional space seems to be very homogeneous; in other words, these transcripts do not form any specific cluster, neither they are attracted to any other given one provided by the transcripts with specific (and unambiguous) relative phase index. The same is true for both studied transcriptomes. Later we discuss this point in more detail, while here we fix that the points representing such multi-CDS transcripts are erased from the pictures illustrating the results.

Thus, the clusters formed by transcripts of the same relative phase index are located in two parallel planes (in the space of three principal components with the largest eigenvalues). This observation holds true for *L. sibirica* transcriptome, while *P. sibirica* transcriptome exhibits some deviations from this pattern. We should discuss it later in more detail.

### 3.2 *L. sibirica* transcriptome octahedron

Unlike the tiles developed for a genome, the transcripts of a transcriptome exhibit an ultimate pattern, that is, octahedron. The rectangular triangles, $\Delta ABC$ and $\Delta\alpha\beta\gamma$, in **Figure 2** occupy the position in two orthogonal planes. Note, these triangles do not comprise the clusters from the same strand; on the contrary, phases over the octahedron are distributed in the manner shown in **Figure 2** (right).

**Figure 3** shows the distribution of *L. sibirica* transcripts with relative phase values ranging from $F_0$ to $B_2$; they are colored as described above. This is the distribution in 63-dimensional space (see Section 2.5.1) shown as the projection into two-dimensional plane determined by the first and the second principal components (**Figure 3**, left) and by the second and the third principal components (**Figure 3**, right); this right image is rotated for $\pi/4$ angle clockwise.

The transcriptome shown in this figure exhibits clear and unambiguous octahedral pattern in cluster location. It is evident that $F_0$ to $F_2$ phases lay out in a plane and vice versa: the phases from the lagging strand are also laid out in a plane, and these two planes are parallel. It should be stressed that this pattern is observed in the metric space defined by the eigenvectors of the covariation matrix; in other words, the clear and apparent octahedron pattern is observed in affinely transformed space, not in the original one determined by triplet frequency.

Let us now consider the distribution of the points corresponding to *noCDS* and *mult* indexes. These two types of sequences differ drastically, in terms of their dispersion over the pattern. The transcripts bearing several CDS (see **Table 1**) are rather long. The distribution of $W_{(3,\,3)}$ of such transcripts is shown in **Figure 4**; it should be stressed that this is the mutual distribution of all the points, with the

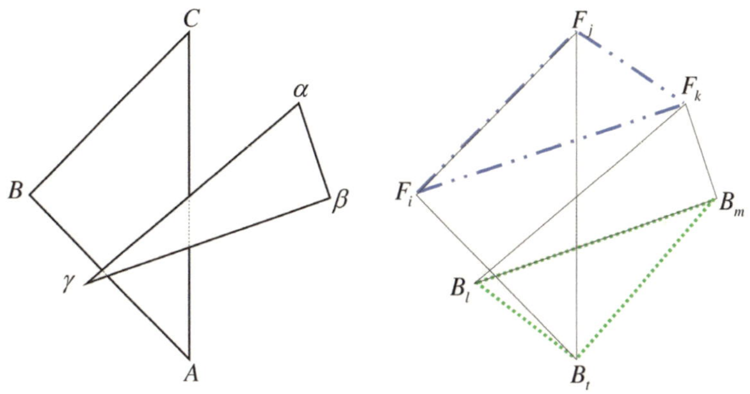


**Figure 2.**
*Typical distribution of L. sibirica transcripts in 63-dimensional space.*

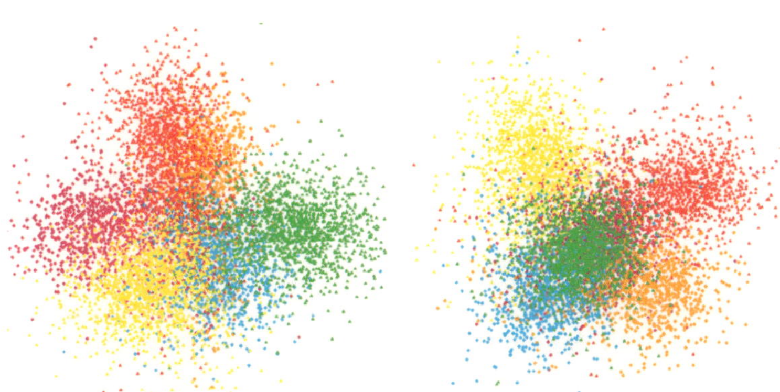

**Figure 3.**
*The distribution of L. sibirica transcripts; phases noCDS and mult are erased.*

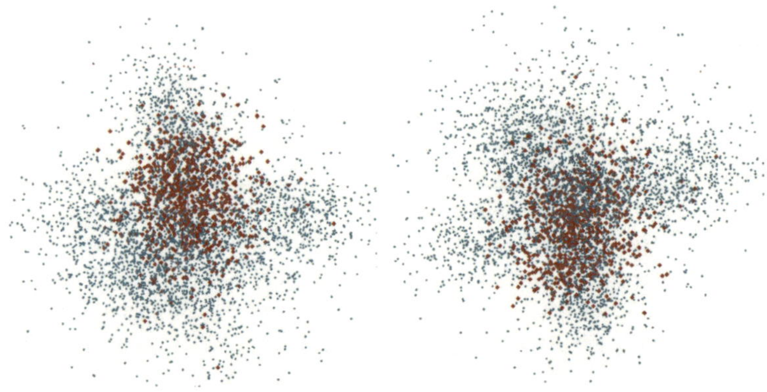

**Figure 4.**
*The distribution of L. sibirica transcripts with noCDS (brown diamonds) and mult sequences (teal circles). The axes are directed in the same way, as in* ***Figure 3****.*

complete set of phase indexes; the only point in this Figure is that the points corresponding to phases $F_0$ through $B_2$ are erased.

Also, this figure shows the distribution of the transcripts where no CDS have been found (brown circles). The cluster comprising these transcripts is rather remarkable: the transcripts where no CDS have been found behave themselves (in terms of clustering in 63-dimensional triplet frequency space) pretty close to the fragments falling completely into noncoding regions of a genome, when a complete genome is sliced into a set of tiles [2–4, 16, 17]. This observation indirectly (while rather hard) proves the total lack of any CDS in such sequences; otherwise, the corresponding frequency dictionaries never could be gathered in a ball centered at the pattern.

The transcripts with several CDS inside are distributed over the pattern almost homogeneously, including the central spot where the transcripts without CDS are concentrated. Apparently, this fact follows from the multiplicity of CDS in these transcripts: an interplay of different CDS located within a transcript may yield an effective value of its *phase* index ranging from $F_0$ to $B_2$, and the impact of those CDS is expected to be rather random.

### 3.3 *P. sibirica* transcriptome octahedron

Let us now focus on the peculiarities of the transcriptome of *P. sibirica*. First of all, this transcriptome (at least, the part taken into analysis) is less abundant, in comparison to *L. sibirica* transcriptome. This fact may impact the pattern of the triplet frequency dictionary distribution, while one may expect the effect to be negligible, since the length distribution of the transcripts of *P. sibirica* is similar to that one observed for *L. sibirica* (see **Figure 1**) and the portion of multi-CDS transcripts in these two transcriptomes are quite similar (see **Table 1**).

To begin with, **Figure 5** shows the clustering pattern observed for this transcriptome; the technology of the development of the pattern is absolutely the same, as in **Figures 3** and 4. The strongest difference between this transcriptome and the *L. sibirica* one consists in the significant deformation of the octahedron observed over *P. sibirica* transcriptome; **Figure 6** illustrates this point.

At the first glance, the pattern shown in **Figure 5** looks like a tetrahedron, while it is not. In proper projection, the pattern looks like a hexagon; adding the subset of multi-CDS transcripts, one gets the same pattern almost homogeneously covered by the point corresponding to the subset.

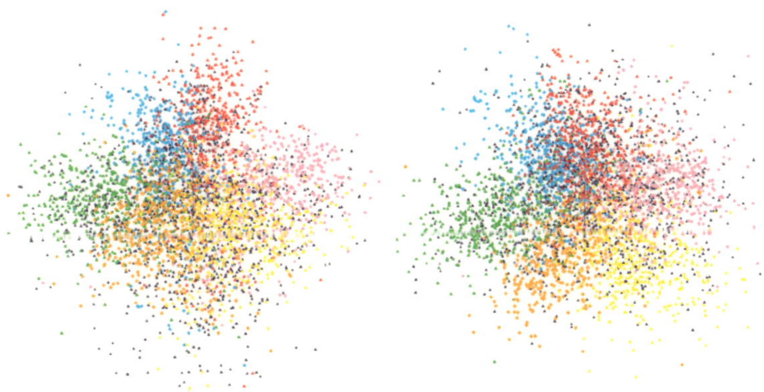

**Figure 5.**
*The distribution of P. sibirica transcripts; the phase mult is erased.*

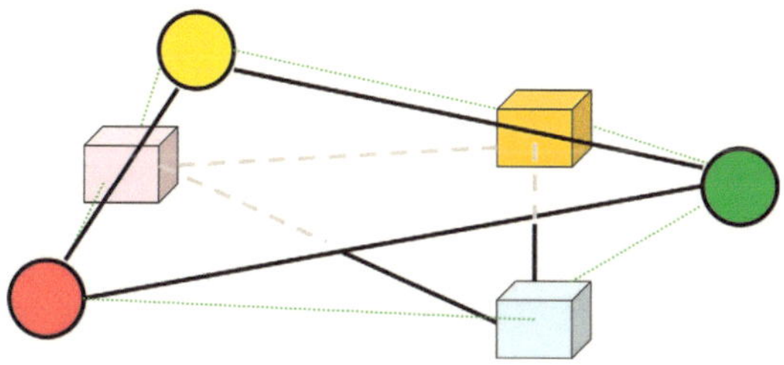

**Figure 6.**
*The deformation of P. sibirica transcriptome. Balls are the clusters of F-strand, and boxes are the clusters of B-strand; coloring follows the layout described above (see Section 3.1).*

## 4. Discussion

The patterns provided by the distribution of considerably short fragments of a genome may tell a lot to a researcher [2–4, 16, 17]. For bacteria, GC content seems to be the key factor determining the details of the pattern [2–4]. That is not so for chloroplasts, mitochondria, and cyanobacteria [16, 17]. The results presented above show that GC content has nothing to do with a pattern observed over a transcriptome. Hence, a question arises toward the key factor determining the specific type of a pattern. Yet, there is no simple and brief answer, while Chargaff's parity rule discrepancy may be quite informative here.

We have determined Chargaff's rule discrepancy measure (5) figure $\mu^{\star}$ for all six clusters observed in *L. sibirica* and *P. sibirica* transcriptomes; **Table 2** shows them. The variation of these figures $\mu^{\star}$ is very smooth, and the clusters are pretty close to each other, in terms of the discrepancy $\mu$ (see Eq. (5)). This fact opposes to similar observations carried out over bacterial, chloroplast, and mitochondrial genomes [16, 17]: these later exhibit significant (more than 10 times) difference in the discrepancy figures calculated for the clusters. It should be said that, unlike transcriptomes, chloroplast genomes exhibit three-beam patterns, where a beam (i.e., a cluster) comprises the fragments from forward and backward strands, simultaneously. There is no such combination, for transcriptomes.

Let us now focus on a few more details on Chargaff's imparity index, itself. The index value differs for different length $q$ of words. Thus, a question arises toward the reference figures for this index. Suppose, the index is determined over the frequency dictionaries derived from both strands; in such capacity, it must be equal to zero.

| | Relative phases | | | | | |
|---|---|---|---|---|---|---|
| **Transcriptome** | $F_0$ | $F_1$ | $F_2$ | $B_0$ | $B_1$ | $B_2$ |
| *L. sibirica* | 0.00129 | 0.00169 | 0.00144 | 0.00160 | 0.00133 | 0.00123 |
| *P. sibirica* | 0.00122 | 0.00154 | 0.00144 | 0.00150 | 0.00135 | 0.00131 |
| *L. sibirica* | 0.12904 | 0.22707 | 0.06629 | 0.06774 | 0.09674 | 0.06201 |
| *P. sibirica* | 0.06944 | 0.07185 | 0.07023 | 0.07163 | 0.07559 | 0.07712 |

**Table 2.**
*Discrepancy measure (5) figures $\mu^{\star}$ for two transcriptomes (upper part) and cluster radii, for the same phases (lower part).*

Calculating the index (4) over a single strand, one may clearly understand to what extend a strand looks like the opposite one, in terms of the word frequency [23–25]. For random non-correlated sequence with $f_A = f_T$ and $f_C = f_G$ $\left(\mu_q = 0\right)$. Hence, $\forall_q.\mu_q$ figures remain the same, if the discrepancy $\mu_1$ is fixed [23].

Unlike $\mu^{\star}$ figures, the radii of these six clusters exhibit quite diverse behavior. The radius of a cluster is an average distance from the center (that is arithmetic mean) determined over the cluster to each point from the cluster. Lower part of **Table 1** shows the radii figures. The radii figures are apparently different, for the transcriptomes under consideration. $F_0$ and $F_1$ phases for *L. sibirica* show extremely high values. These figures may not be explained by the excess of the cluster abundance of *L. sibirica* in comparison to *P. sibirica*. Again, the variation of the radii for *L. sibirica* is evidently greater than for *P. sibirica*, and this fact correlates to the mirror symmetry of *P. sibirica* transcriptome, since it is typical for simpler and less diverse genetic system.

Inter-cluster discrepancy measure $\mu$ is of great interest, for both cases; **Table 3** shows these indexes. Careful examination of **Table 3** allows to identify three couples of relative phase indexes with distinctively lower figure of (4), namely, the couples:

$$F_0 \Leftrightarrow B_2 \qquad F_1 \Leftrightarrow B_0 \qquad F_2 \Leftrightarrow B_1. \tag{6}$$

| | | | *L. sibirica* | | |
|---|---|---|---|---|---|
| **Phase index** | $F_1$ | $F_2$ | $B_0$ | $B_1$ | $B_2$ |
| $F_0$ | 0.00095 | 0.00111 | 0.00098 | 0.00101 | 0.00007 |
| $F_1$ | | 0.00094 | 0.00008 | 0.00109 | 0.00102 |
| $F_2$ | | | 0.00111 | 0.00009 | 0.00105 |
| $B_0$ | | | | 0.00090 | 0.00090 |
| $B_1$ | | | | | 0.00105 |
| | | | ***P. sibirica*** | | |
| $F_0$ | 0.00091 | 0.00105 | 0.00096 | 0.00028 | 0.00099 |
| $F_1$ | | 0.00094 | 0.00008 | 0.00107 | 0.00105 |
| $F_2$ | | | 0.00112 | 0.00110 | 0.00016 |
| $B_0$ | | | | 0.00098 | 0.00087 |
| $B_1$ | | | | | 0.00105 |

**Table 3.**
*Discrepancy measure (4) figures $\mu$ determined within each of the two transcriptomes.*

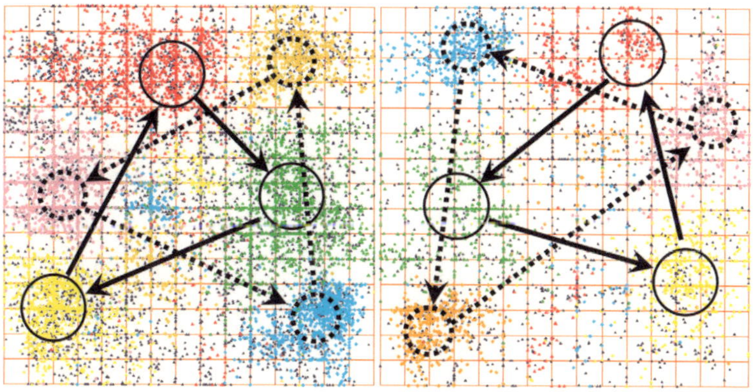

**Figure 7.**
*Mirror (left) symmetry in L. sibirica transcriptome vs. shift symmetry (right) in P. sibirica transcriptome. Solid circles and solid arrows correspond to F phases, while dashed ones correspond to B phases.*

Evidently, the phases in these couples yield two different types of symmetry: the first one is shift, and the second symmetry is mirror. The situation is opposite for *P. sibirica* transcriptome: the couples with the least Chargaff's discrepancy measure (4) are the following:

$$F_0 \Leftrightarrow B_1 \qquad F_1 \Leftrightarrow B_0 \qquad F_2 \Leftrightarrow B_2. \tag{7}$$

To make the situation with symmetries clear, we show the clusters over the elastic map shown in the so-called *inner coordinates*; **Figure 7** presents the transcriptomes.

Such mirror symmetry has been previously reported for chloroplast genomes [16, 17] (see also [23, 37, 38]); yet, there were no other but the chloroplast genomes exhibiting such mirror symmetry, and *L. sibirica* transcriptome is the next one in this point.

Definitely, the coincidence of these two symmetrical patterns does not mean that *L. sibirica* transcriptome is identical to a chloroplast genome in all other properties. Probably, plants differ from other eukaryotic organisms and bacteria in the symmetry type; currently, no eukaryotic genome is found with mirror symmetry. Shift symmetry observed for *P. sibirica* transcriptome poses a question toward the origin of the symmetry type change: whether it results from some essential biological difference between these two pine species or it is a manifestation of the genomic transformation in witch's broom cells. To answer the question, more studies are necessary.

The most amazing thing in transcriptome statistical properties is that it yields an octahedral pattern, unlike bacteria, organelle, and other genetic entities (say, yeast genomes). Another point is that the pattern does not depend on the length of transcripts taken into consideration: we have examined separately the subsets of transcripts as long as $200 \le N \le 600$ bp, $600 \le N \le 2500$ bp, and those longer 3000 bp. All these subsets yield similar pattern, with very minor variation mainly manifesting in cluster density.

One can easily see two major peculiarities differing a transcriptome from the sets of tiles described above (see [2–4, 16, 17] for details). These are:

- Total absence of the (rather extended) noncoding regions.
- Elimination of introns from the statistical analysis of sequences.

Of course, the first item from this list is quite arguable: a number of transcripts where no CDS has been detected bring a direct and unambiguous disproof of it. Thus, the question arises, whether these transcripts are similar, in some sense, to the fragments of genome comprising purely noncoding regions of the latter.

We have examined the first hypothesis through the simulation of noncoding regions. To do that, we have added a number of $W_{(3,\ 3)}$ frequency dictionaries obtained from the tiles covering the noncoding parts of genomes of several other organisms. All the tiles were as long as 603 bp and contained noncoding regions, exclusively. The number of dictionaries (the points, in other words) varied from one third to one half of the total number of transcripts in the set. By assumption, this addition simulated a genome.

Upon addition, we expected to see a pattern similar to that one observed in bacteria, organelle, or other eukaryotic organisms; the octahedron pattern appeared to be stronger. **Figure 8** obviously disproves this hypothesis: it shows the same transcriptome (*L. sibirica*) with eliminated transcripts bearing no CDS, where a set of $W_{(3,\ 3)}$ dictionaries borrowed from three different genomes is added,

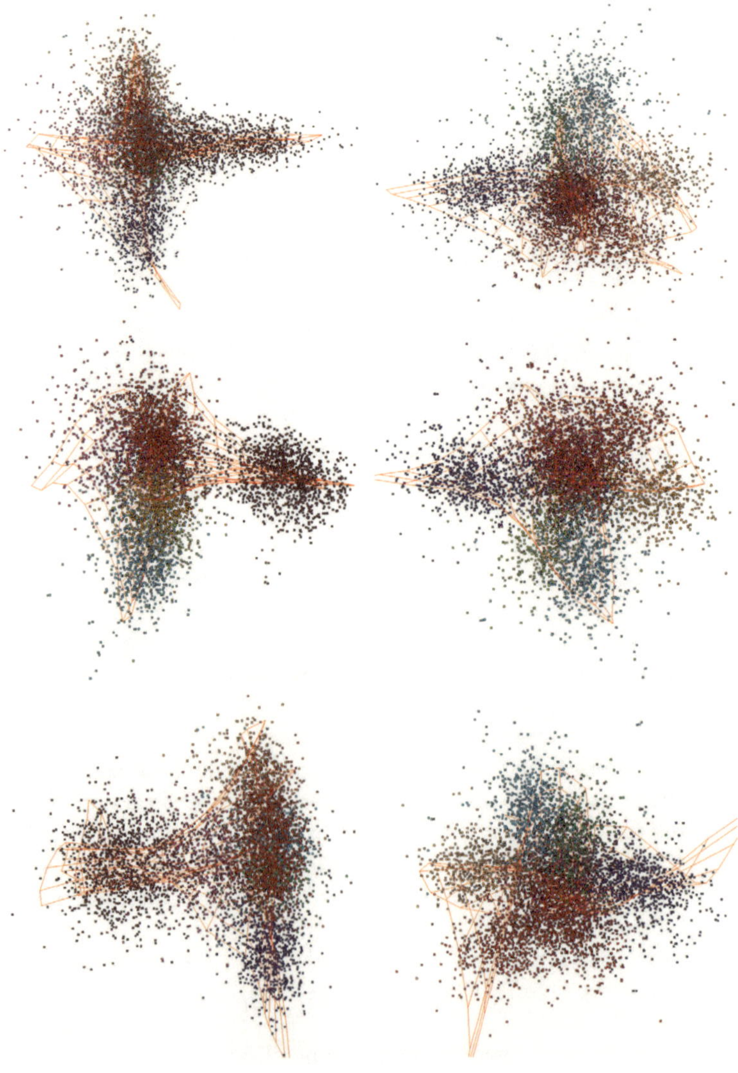

**Figure 8.**
*Three noncoding data points added to L. sibirica transcriptome; nothing happened.*

consequently. Obviously, such simulation of a genome does not break down the observed pattern of transcript distribution. Yet, one more option should be examined: what happens if the natural noncoding regions are used to simulate a genome? In other words, the pattern might be sensitive to the noncoding regions from the original genome, only, This point still awaits for examination.

The impact of introns on the alteration of the observed pattern is less evident. Moreover, one faces greater difficulties in revealing it. One might want to compare the distributions developed over $W_{(3,\ 3)}$ and $W_3$ dictionaries, in this case; yet, this problem needs careful investigation and falls beyond the scope of this paper.

## 5. Conclusions

Systematic comparison of (rather short) fragments of permanent length formally identified within a genome reveals a symmetry in the distribution of the triplet frequency dictionaries obtained over those fragments; originally this effect has been found on bacterial genomes. Later similar (while rather different in a number of essential details) behavior has been found for chloroplasts and mitochondria genomes. The general pattern of the distribution looks like a superposition of two triangles where the vertices correspond to the fragments of the same relative phase. In simple words, it corresponds to a reading frame shift, in case of a translation-like processing of DNA sequence.

A transcriptome itself might be considered as a set of those fragments, with few exclusions. Firstly, the lengths of transcripts are different and may affect the expected pattern. Secondly, there are no fragments in a transcriptome corresponding to those obtained from noncoding (intergenic) regions of a genome. This fact results in ultimate possible configuration of the clusters corresponding to the transcripts with the same relative phase index, that is, octahedron. All these patterns could be seen in the space of three principal components with the largest eigenvalues. The *L. sibirica* transcriptome yields almost perfect octahedral pattern, while the *P. sibirica* transcriptome differs rather significantly, with planes comprising the clusters from the same strand to be located almost in parallel. This deformation might result from the biology: we studied the *P. sibirica* transcriptome obtained not from a normal tree, but from a witch's broom bud; the latter is known for extremely deviated morphology that may not avoid serious genetic alteration in its genome.

## Acknowledgements

The data used in this study were obtained under the grant 14.Y26.31.0004 from the Russian Government. The authors also thank Serafima Novikova from Siberian Federal University for the helpful discussion.

## Conflict of interest

The authors declare no conflict of interest.

## Author details

Sadovsky Michael[1,2*], Putintseva Yulia[2], Biryukov Vladislav[2] and Senashova Maria[1]

1 Institute of Computational Modeling SB RAS, Krasnoyarsk, Russia

2 Siberian Federal University, Institute of Fundamental Biology and Biotechnology, Krasnoyarsk, Russia

*Address all correspondence to: msad@icm.krasn.ru

## References

[1] Weiss LE, Naor T, Shechtman Y. Observing DNA in live cells. Biochemical Society Transactions. 2018; **46**(3):729-740

[2] Gorban AN, Popova TG, Zinovyev AY. Codon usage trajectories and 7-cluster structure of 143 complete bacterial genomic sequences. Physica A: Statistical Mechanics and its Applications. 2005;**353**:365-387

[3] Gorban AN, Popova TG, Zinovyev AY. Seven clusters in genomic triplet distributions. In Silico Biology. 2003;**3**(4):471-482

[4] Gorban AN, Popova TG, Zinovyev AY. Four basic symmetry types in the universal 7-cluster structure of microbial genomic sequences. In Silico Biology. 2005;**5**(3):265-282

[5] Chu KH, Qi J, Yu ZG, Anh V. Origin and phylogeny of chloroplasts revealed by a simple correlation analysis of complete genomes. Molecular Biology and Evolution. 2004;**1**:200-206

[6] Tsiligaridis J. Multiple sequence alignment and clustering with dot matrices, entropy, and genetic algorithms. In: Li K-C, Jiang H, Yang LT, Cuzzocreapp A, editors. Chapter 4 in Big Data: Algorithms, Analytics, and Applications. CRC Press; 2015. pp. 71-88

[7] Znamenskij SV. Modeling of the optimal sequence alignment problem. Program Systems: Theory and Applications. 2014;**4**(22):257-267 (in Russian)

[8] Znamenskij SV. A model and algorithm for sequence alignment. Program Systems: Theory and Applications. 2015;**1**(24):189-197

[9] Antipov D, Raiko M, Lapidus A, Pevzner PA. Plasmid detection and assembly in genomic and metagenomic datasets. Genome Research. 2019;**26**(9): 961-968

[10] Vignesh U, Parvathi R. Biological Big Data analysis and visualization: A survey. In: Biotechnology: Concepts, Methodologies, Tools, and Applications. IGI Global; 2019. pp. 653-665

[11] Kaur S, Kaur S, Sood SK. Proposed better sequence alignment for identification of organisms using DNA barcode. In: Innovations in Computational Intelligence. Singapore: Springer; 2018. pp. 115-150

[12] Bugaenko NN, Gorban AN, Sadovsky MG. Towards the definition of information content of nucleotide sequences. Molecular Biology. 1996; **30**(5):529-541 (in Russian)

[13] Bugaenko NN, Gorban AN, Sadovsky MG. The information capacity of nucleotide sequences and their fragments. Biophysics. 1997;**5**: 1063-1069 (in Russian)

[14] Bugaenko NN, Gorban AN, Sadovsky MG. Maximum entropy method in analysis of genetic text and measurement of its information content. Open Systems and Information Dynamics. 1998;**5**(2):265-278

[15] Hu R, Wang B. Statistically significant strings are related to regulatory elements in the promoter regions of *Saccharomyces cerevisiae*. Physica A: Statistical Mechanics and its Applications. 2001;**290**:464-474

[16] Sadovsky MG, Senashova MY, Malyshev AV. Chloroplast genomes exhibit eight-cluster structuredness and mirror symmetry. In: Rojas I, Ortuño F, editors. Bioinformatics and Biomedical Engineering. Cham: Springer International Publishing; 2018. pp. 186-196. LNBI 10813

[17] Sadovsky MG, Senashova MY, Putintseva YA. Chapter 2. Eight clusters, synchrony of evolution and unique symmetry in chloroplast genomes: The offering from triplets. In: Chloroplasts and Cytoplasm: Structure and Functions. Nova Science Publishers, Inc.; 2018. pp. 25-95

[18] Krutovsky KV, Oreshkova NV, Putintseva YA, Ibe AA, Deich KO, Shilkina EA. Preliminary results of *de novo* whole genome sequencing of Siberian larch (*Larix sibirica* Ledeb.) and Siberian stone pine (*Pinus sibirica* Du Tour.). Siberian Journal of Forest Science. 2014;**1**(4):79-83

[19] Oreshkova NV, Putintseva YA, Kuzmin DA, Sharov VV, Biryukov VV, Makolov SV, et al. Genome sequencing and assembly of Siberian larch (*Larix sibirica* Ledeb.) and Siberian pine (*Pinus sibirica* Du Tour) and preliminary transcriptome data. In: Proceedings of the 4th International Conference on Conservation of Forest Genetic Resources in Siberia, August 24-29, 2015, Barnaul: Barnaul State university; 2015. pp. 127-128

[20] Fukunaga K. Introduction to Statistical Pattern Recognition. Vol. 625. London, Berlin, Heidelberg: Academic Press; 1990

[21] Elson D, Chargaff E. On the deoxyribonucleic acid content of sea urchin gametes. Experientia. 1952;**8**(4): 143-145

[22] Chargaff E, Lipshitz R, Green C. Composition of the deoxypentose nucleic acids of four genera of sea-urchin. The Journal of Biological Chemistry. 1952;**195**(1):155-160

[23] Grebnev YV, Sadovsky MG. Chargaff's second rule and symmetry in genomes. Fundamental Studies. 2014; **12**(5):965-968 (in Russian)

[24] Sánchez J, José MV. Analysis of bilateral inverse symmetry in whole bacterial chromosomes. Biochemical and Biophysical Research Communications. 2002;**299**(1):126-134

[25] Mitchell D, Bridge R. A test of Chargaff's second rule. Biochemical and Biophysical Research Communications. 2006;**340**(1):90-94

[26] Afreixo V, Bastos CAC, Garcia SP, Rodrigues JMOS, Pinho AJ, Ferreira PJSG. The breakdown of the word symmetry in the human genome. Journal of Theoretical Biology. 2013;**335**: 153-159

[27] Touchon M, Rocha EPC. From GC skews to wavelets: A gentle guide to the analysis of compositional asymmetries in genomic data. Biochimie. 2008; **90**(4):648-659

[28] Mascher M, Schubert I, Scholz U, Friedel S. Patterns of nucleotide asymmetries in plant and animal genomes. Bio Systems. 2013;**111**(3):181-189

[29] Bultrini E, Pizzi E, Del Giudice P, Frontali C. Pentamer vocabularies characterizing introns and intron-like intergenic tracts from *Caenorhabditis elegans* and *Drosophila melanogaster*. Gene. 2003;**304**:183-192

[30] Nikolaou C, Almirantis Y. Deviations from Chargaff's second parity rule in organellar DNA: Insights into the evolution of organellar genomes. Gene. 2006;**381**:34-41

[31] Frank AC, Lobry JR. Asymmetric substitution patterns: A review of possible underlying mutational or selective mechanisms. Gene. 1999;**238**(1):65-77

[32] Guo FB, Yu XJ. Separate base usages of genes located on the leading and lagging strands in *Chlamydia muridarum* revealed by the Z curve method. BMC Genomics. 2007;**8**(1):366

[33] Nikolaou C, Almirantis Y. Mutually symmetric and complementary triplets:

Differences in their use distinguish systematically between coding and non-coding genomic sequences. Journal of Theoretical Biology. 2003;**223**(4): 477-487

[34] Bansal M. DNA structure: Revisiting the Watson-Crick double helix. Current Science. 2003;**85**(11):1556-1563

[35] Mandoiu I, Zelikovsky A. Bioinformatics Algorithms: Techniques and Applications. Vol. 3. John Wiley & Sons; 2008

[36] De Fonzo V, Aluffi-Pentini F, Parisi V. Hidden Markov models in bioinformatics. Current Bioinformatics. 2007;**2**(1):49-61

[37] Niu DK, Lin K, Zhang DY. Strand compositional asymmetries of nuclear DNA in eukaryotes. Jouranl of Molecular Evolution. 2003;**57**(3): 325-334

[38] Qu H, Wu H, Zhang T, Zhang Z, Hu S, Yu J. Nucleotide compositional asymmetry between the leading and lagging strands of eubacterial genomes. Research in Microbiology. 2010;**161**: 838-846